ORTHOPAEDIC PROBLEMS
AT WORK

by M. LAURENS ROWE, M.D.

Consultant in Orthopaedic Surgery
Eastman Kodak Company (retired)
Chief Emeritus, Orthopaedic Surgery
Rochester General Hospital
Associate Clinical Professor, Orthopaedic Surgery
University of Rochester School of Medicine
Rochester, New York

CONTENTS

LIST OF ILLUSTRATIONS AND TABLES

iv

INTRODUCTION

About half of all Workers' Compensation cases involve musculo-skeletal conditions which technically lie within the designated domain of orthopaedics. The majority are relatively minor problems which are treated on an ambulatory basis by industrial physicians and nurses, emergency room personnel or family doctors. Most never come under the care of orthopaedic surgeons.

Even minor orthopaedic problems, however, frequently result in some degree of permanent partial disability, at least as defined by the schedules of the various State Workers' Compensation Laws. Usually the permanency is mild but, because of the large number of cases, aggregate awards can be significant. Residual disability can be reduced in many cases by more knowledgeable early treatment.

More importantly, a number of conditions notorious for producing severe disability masquerade, in the beginning, as minor problems seemingly amenable to ambulatory dispensary treatment. Early identification of these conditions, recognition of their threat, and immediate referral for expert care can materially reduce lost time and permanency.

Relatively little teaching time is allotted to common minor ortho-paedic problems in the typical crowded medical school curriculum and there may be no opportunity for physicians to acquire expertise in the management of these conditions during internship and residency training. Consequently, many primary care physicians in industry and in private or clinic practice may have to undertake the treatment of patients with minor musculo-skeletal problems with but rudimentary knowledge of the subject.

Textbooks of Orthopaedic Surgery deal mainly with major musculo-skeletal problems requiring hospital care and surgical treatment and there is a dearth of ready information on the care and management of the minor orthopaedic conditions which constitute such a large share of the industrial medical work load. There is a need for a concise manual on the treatment of common minor musculo-skeletal problems at work directed toward the non-orthopaedically trained occupational physicians and nurses who daily encounter them.

In order to identify the most common orthopaedic problem in industrial practice and aid in the choice and focus of the subject material, a thousand consecutive orthopaedic cases reported to the

1

Workers' Compensation Board by a large industry were tabulated by anatomical area and diagnosis. Their anatomical distribution is shown on the body map in Figure 1.

Throughout the book, a number in parentheses after each anatomical area indicates the number of cases involving that area. Each clinical entity within the anatomical region is similarly designated by a numerical indication of incidence of that condition in the thousand case sampling. This Frequency Index not only conveys some notion as to the rate of occurrence of a given diagnosis but also helps to insure that appropriate attention is devoted in the text to the common conditions most often treated by occupational physicians and nurses.

Text material is arranged according to an anatomical outline with a separate chapter devoted to each body region. Within each region, clinical entities are presented by diagnosis. An introduction to each chapter describes the structural, functional and pathomechanical features of the anatomical region which foretell the kinds of clinical conditions likely to occur and determine general principles of treatment.

Conditions for which specialist treatment is obviously indicated are identified but are not discussed in detail apart from diagnosis and suggestions for emergency care. A few conditions not encountered in the thousand case sample are included and indicated by an asterisk rather than a Frequency Index designation. Some are common orthopaedic conditions seen among workers but not often reported as compensation cases. Others are injuries which appear innocuous but which threaten severe disability and require expert care.

Certain special considerations are peculiar to the management of orthopaedic problems at work. Patients are commonly seen much sooner after injury or the onset of symptoms than is usual in the outside practice of orthopaedics. Slightly different approaches in history taking and some special techniques in examination are useful. An expanded concept of injury becomes pertinent. General tissue responses to trauma govern the early stages of treatment and are important to review. Patient management may be complicated by an adversary situation between employee and employer which sometimes develops in Workers' Compensation cases. These and similar considerations peculiar to Industrial Orthopaedics are discussed in a separate opening chapter.

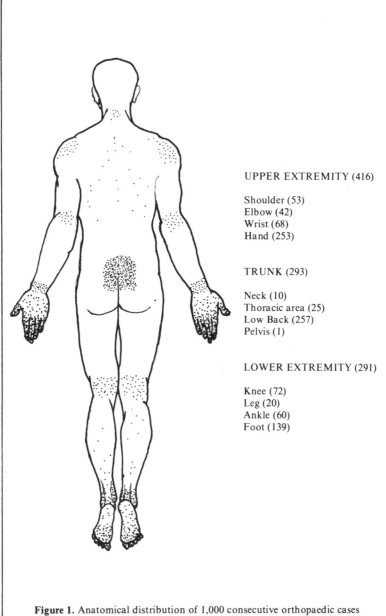

UPPER EXTREMITY (416)

Shoulder (53)
Elbow (42)
Wrist (68)
Hand (253)

TRUNK (293)

Neck (10)
Thoracic area (25)
Low Back (257)
Pelvis (1)

LOWER EXTREMITY (291)

Knee (72)
Leg (20)
Ankle (60)
Foot (139)

Figure 1. Anatomical distribution of 1,000 consecutive orthopaedic cases reported to the Workers' Compensation Board as on-the-job injuries or work-related conditions.

CHAPTER 1
SPECIAL CONSIDERATIONS IN
INDUSTRIAL ORTHOPAEDICS

Competent management of patients with musculo-skeletal problems in industry may require sharpening of some of the therapist's professional skills, review and up-dating of anatomy and of the pathology of trauma, and revision of some ideas concerning injury and the Workers' Compensation process. The special considerations which enter into the treatment of orthopaedic cases in the workplace can be summarized under six main headings:
1. Expanded concept of injury
2. The influence of Workers' Compensation Laws
3. History taking in work-related complaints
4. Special examination techniques
5. Traumatology
6. Regional orthopaedic principles

THE MANY FACES OF INJURY
Injury, in one of its several guises, enters into diagnostic consideration in virtually every patient in industry who presents with musculo-skeletal complaints.

In its simplest form, it is the single accident in which clearly defined trauma is sustained by a previously well individual and which results in a predictable degree and duration of disability. The exact time, date and circumstances of the injury can be established, the nature and extent of the tissue damage is consistent with the degree and type of trauma, and the injury constitutes the sole and competent cause of the disability.

In less clear-cut form, it is the muscle pain which follows a period of unaccustomed heavy work, usually after a lag phase, typically upon getting out of bed the next morning. No single moment of injury can be defined and, usually, there are no immediate symptoms to indicate that injury has occurred. Furthermore, the same amount of physical activity would not cause symptoms in all individuals, nor even in the same individual at a different time when appropriate physical conditioning

5

for the task would probably prevent the reaction. An element of host susceptibility has been introduced into the injury equation. In this case, it is lack of conditioning, a susceptibility factor which is reversible.

In a still more subtle manifestation, it is the tendon pain which may occur in certain individuals after engaging in highly repetitive but not necessarily very stressful activity. Again, there is no single moment of injury and, as in the instance above, exposure to the same amount of repetitive activity will not produce symptoms in all individuals. Again, there is an element of individual susceptibility. This time, however, the susceptibility is much less likely to be reversible. Certain individuals, for reasons that are neither well understood nor identifiable in advance, will respond repeatedly with tendon pain upon exposure to highly repetitive work. Symptoms are due to an inflammatory reaction in the tendon sheath (tenosynovitis) and the injury of repetitive activity is generally accepted as the proximate, if not the only, cause of the disability.

In yet another guise of injury, an accidental incident which is relatively trivial leads to an extended period of unexpectedly severe disability because of pre-existing changes in the involved tissues. A patient with degenerative arthritis of the knee, often heretofore unrecognized, sustains a minor bump or twist of the knee, develops massive swelling and severe pain out of all proportion to the degree of injury, and may have protracted disability. The same degree of trauma might be inconsequential in the individual with a normal joint. In Workers' Compensation parlance, this is termed "aggravation of a pre-existing condition" and is accepted as a fairly common variant of the injury process.

Certain conditions, especially in the low back, may give rise to spontaneous episodes of pain which can occur suddenly in the course of normal activity without any definable accident or recognizable trauma. This may be the most confusing and vexing manifestation of the injury process with which to cope. Most Workers' Compensation laws provide that, when symptoms appear while the patient is at work, the case is reportable as compensable injury since it arises "out of and in the course of employment."

Whether such cases are actually reported as compensable injury often depends upon factors which have little to do with injury or with the medical condition. The patient who has done heavy work for years is more likely to be reported on the unproved assumption that the long period of hard labor may have caused the condition in the low back and because the symptoms will likely produce more disability than they would in the sedentary worker. The desk worker whose pain occurs while reaching for a paper clip is less likely to be reported, although the legal claim for such recourse may be equally valid.

In actuality, it may be the patient who determines whether the case is reported as compensable injury simply by the manner in which the history is recited. The patient who has had many previous similar episodes, both at home and at work, is less likely to claim causal relationship to the job. On the other hand, the patient with a first attack of low back pain may relate the symptoms to work activity, as may the patient with a poor work record, job dissatisfaction and an eye to secondary gain.

All of the many manifestations of the injury process must be interpreted with recognition of the normal universal tendency to attribute all musculo-skeletal symptoms to mechanical forces until conclusively proved otherwise. The magnitude and immediacy of trauma is generally overstated by patients with these kinds of symptoms, not necessarily with any attempt to defraud.

The occupational physician or nurse must exercise perceptive judgement as to the true significance of injury as either sole or contributing cause of symptoms. Upon this initial judgement often rests the outcome of the management of the case.

WORKERS' COMPENSATION AND
INDUSTRIAL ORTHOPAEDICS

Prior to the adoption of the first Workers' Compensation law in 1910, the worker was presumed to be a free agent, voluntarily taking a job and thereby assuming whatever risks were inherent in the job. The only recourse for injury at work was to sue the employer, a step which, given the limited resources of the average worker, was unlikely to succeed. Thousands of workers' families were left destitute by work accidents and there was mounting social protest. Workers' Compensation legislation was aimed at redressing this social injustice. The system favors the worker and places liability solely upon the employer. Fault and negligence are immaterial. Workers' Compensation legislation created laws of social welfare and, like much legislation seeking to correct evils on one side, may have created evils on the other.

Many claims of work injury appear unjust. The legal definition of compensable injury is extremely broad and often at variance with traditional medical definitions. Decision as to whether a case is reported as compensable frequently seems capricious and arbitrary.

Attuned to laws of justice rather than those of social welfare and generally only vaguely aware of the background of Workers' Compensation legislation, it is easy for loyal Company people at the work site, in the medical department and even in the Workers' Compensation office to adopt judgemental attitudes with regard to claims of work injury. To the extent that they transmit their attitudes to the patient, they may be instrumental in creating bitter adversary relationships between employee and employer which can affect the outcome of treatment and prolong and maximize the disability. Experienced occupational physicians and nurses will leave judgement to the Workers' Compensation Referees and the laws in the hands of their elected legislators. The patient is best served by those who understand and make allowances for the intent and nature of Workers' Compensation laws and hold themselves free of judgemental or adversary roles.

HISTORY TAKING

A detailed and accurate description of the presenting complaint and its time and mode of onset is of prime importance in industrial orthopaedics. There will usually be a history of injury. It then becomes the task of the interviewer to develop a sufficiently clear picture of the injury to determine whether it, alone, constitutes adequate cause for symptoms; whether it is capable of aggravating a pre-existing condition; or whether it is a retrospective concept on the part of the patient to explain musculo-skeletal symptoms. It may be necessary to interview witnesses in order to reconstruct the incident and reach a firm decision.

The first history is usually the best history. It is often the occupational nurse who sees the patient first and who has the best opportunity to obtain the most valid information upon which to base judgement. A complete and accurate history has been said by wise clinicians to be 75 percent of the diagnosis.

Table I shows a suggested outline for an industrial orthopaedic history.

PHYSICAL EXAMINATION

Minor modifications in standard examination techniques and painstaking medical record keeping are important elements in the successful management of workers with musculo-skeletal conditions. Patients in industry are usually seen within minutes or a very few hours after the onset of symptoms. Early physical findings often have unique diagnostic

OUTLINE FOR INDUSTRIAL ORTHOPAEDIC HISTORY
I. Presenting Complaint
 A. Complete and accurate description. Patient's words in quotes.
 B. If extremity, double check whether right or left and make sure all entries in the record are consistent.
 C. Mode of onset
  1. Sudden or gradual?
  2. Associated with single injury? Unaccustomed activity? Repetitive motion? Sudden pressure or temperature change?
  3. If associated with injury
   a. Detailed description (time, date, circumstances)
   b. Immediate effects? (deformity, swelling, discoloration, loss of function)
   c. If symptoms delayed, time and circumstances of onset
 D. Progress of condition since onset
 E. Effect of treatment, if any
  1. Local heat or cold application? Medication? Manipulation?
  2. Mobilization versus immobilization?
  3. Best position for comfort? Worst?

II. Past History
 A. Similar symptoms in past? When? Circumstances?
 B. Other musculo-skeletal symptoms? (contralateral area, arthritic, bursitic, rheumatic symptoms)

III. Family History (parents and siblings)
 A. Condition similar to patient's?
 B. Arthritis, bursitis, rheumatism, gout?
 C. Congenital musculo-skeletal defects?

IV. Socio-Economic History
 A. Kind of work? Work record? Time on same job? Relationships in department? Job satisfaction?
 B. Evidence of adaptive resilience (medical record)
  1. Frequency of visits? Lost time? Frequency and duration appropriate to medical condition?
  2. Level of complaints versus objective findings in past?
  3. Home and family situation?
 C. Possible significance of present complaints in above areas?

Table I. A suggested outline for history taking in orthopaedic problems at work.

significance, but they may be evanescent and their value lost unless they are carefully recorded. Because of shift work and other scheduling problems, the worker-patient may be seen by several different therapists during the course of treatment. The medical record, quite apart from its real or potential legal significance, must be an adequate medium of communication between therapists.

This implies more detailed (and more legible) entries than are the norm for the average private office record. Abbreviations which may be crystal clear to one examiner may be totally meaningless to the next. Wherever possible, findings should be expressed numerically by actual measurement: the diameter of a discolored area in inches or centimeters; the loss of motion of a joint in degrees; the amount of swelling of an area in inches or centimeters difference in circumference as compared with the opposite normal area. The tape measure and the small plastic goniometer should be standard pocket equipment for the occupational physician or nurse dealing with orthopaedic problems at work.

Negative Findings

Negative findings on original examination may be as important as positive ones. The ability of a patient actively to flex or extend a joint completely when seen soon after injury may exclude a diagnosis of tendon rupture even though, later on, that ability may be lost because of pain, swelling and muscle spasm. Failure by the early examiner to record the negative finding could easily lead to later doubt in diagnosis, the possible need for surgical exploration, needless prolongation of the recovery period and an increase in the final degree of disability.

Symptom patterns may change in the days following trauma. A hip injury associated with pain on motion of the joint may, with the passage of time, produce severe knee pain while the original hip symptoms may fade and even disappear. Recorded evidence by the original examiner that the knee was normal immediately following the injury may be of prime importance, not only in the medical management of the case, but in protecting the employer from an unwarranted claim of injury to the knee. Negative findings in areas adjoining the site of injury and those which could conceivably be affected by the traumatic incident or by common pain referral patterns should be rountinely recorded.

Point of Tenderness

In addition to the customary description of the symptomatic area in terms of swelling, discoloration, deformity, temperature change and functional loss, accurate recording of the point or points of maximum tenderness should be routine. This valuable information is often available only to the early examiner. With the passage of time following injury, tender spots become diffused and the opportunity for an exact anatomical diagnosis may be lost. Shifting points or areas of tenderness in the days following trauma or the onset of symptoms may also have diagnostic significance, but can be recognized only if the early findings are accurately recorded. Rubber stamp diagrams of anatomical areas are available and may be helpful in indicating points of tenderness.

Comparison With the Contralateral

Comparison of the injured or symptomatic extremity part with the opposite normal area is always useful. What is at first thought to be deformity or instability of an injured joint may turn out, on comparison with the opposite uninjured joint, to be normal for the patient. Wide individual differences in the range of motion of joints, the configuration of extremities and the degree of ligamentous tightness or laxity are common, and the only normal standard for each patient is the opposite unaffected extremity.

Range of Motion of Joints

Transmission of information regarding the range of motion of joints via the medical record is often confusing. Two methods of recording range of motion are in common use. One, recommended by the American Academy of Orthopaedic Surgeons, denotes the fully extended position of a joint as 0 degrees. The other indicates full extension as 180 degrees. In the knee, for instance, the AAOS notation for normal range of motion would be from 0 degrees (full extension) to 135 degrees (full flexion). The second method would describe the same range of motion as progressing from 180 degrees (full extension) to 45 degrees (full flexion). With either method of reporting, the knee has traversed through a range of motion of 135 degrees.

A more meaningful and less confusing method of recording limitation of motion, which is really the point of interest, is to measure, in degrees, the maximum angles of extension and of flexion of the opposite normal joint, using either method. Then perform the same measurements on the injured joint, using the same method. Record the number of degrees of restricted motion in extension and in flexion in the injured joint. "The injured right knee shows a loss of the terminal 15 degrees of extension and 45 degrees of flexion as compared with the uninjured left knee." This conveys the essential information and, at the same time, takes into account the normal standard for each individual patient, the contra-lateral joint.

Circumference Measurements

Measurement of the circumference of extremities objectify the degree of joint or soft tissue swelling and permit accurate estimation of the progress under treatment or observation. Such measurements are easily and quickly made by passing a tape around each extremity perpendicular to its long axis and at corresponding levels in the two extremities. Similar levels can be selected by measuring upward or downward a similar distance from any convenient bony landmark in an uninvolved area of the extremity and using a skin mark to indicate the level of circumferential measurement. The dominant side extremity will norm-ally measure about ¼ inch larger in circumference than the nondominant side.

Comparative circumference measurements may also help to quantitate the degree of disability in the patient with chronic musculo-skeletal complaints. For example, a complaint of severe pain and disability of the knee of more than a few week's duration, unaccompanied by measurable atrophy of the thigh, suggests insignificant objective abnormality of the knee.

X-Rays

X-rays are almost always indicated in acute injury situations but frequently unnecessary views are taken because of failure of the examiner to indicate the exact area of injury on the x-ray requisition. An ink mark on the skin overlying the point of maximum tenderness will often result in a more helpful x-ray examination with fewer exposures.

The examiner should be familiar with the various special x-ray views available for best visualization of specific anatomical areas and injuries and order these views in addition to the routine x-ray examination where they are indicated.

As in the clinical examination, comparison x-rays of the opposite uninjured part may be of critical value in reaching an accurate diagnosis.

GENERAL TRAUMATOLOGY

Certain features of acute injury are common to all anatomical areas and can be considered in a general fashion. Fractures, dislocations, sprains, strains and contusions all produce tissue damage resulting in the exudation of blood and serum into the area of trauma. Swelling and discoloration are the clinical manifestations of this internal oozing. The natural processes of repair begin after the hemorrhagic and serum exudate has been absorbed.

Repair will proceed more rapidly and disability time will be minimized if early steps are taken to limit the exudation of blood and serum into the tissues. This is done by the immediate application of cold, compression and elevation. Heat is not used in the early treatment of acute injury since it produces vasodilatation and increases the oozing of blood and serum into the traumatized area.

Cold may be applied in the form of ice packs made by filling plastic bags with crushed ice or by means of commercially available chemical cold packs. Both should be wrapped in fabric to prevent frost-bite from direct contact of ice or chemical cold with the skin. Lacking ice or chemical packs, cold water may be used except that it usually requires a dependent position of the injured part and is difficult to combine with compression and elevation.

Compression is ordinarily obtained by the use of elastic bandages which may be wrapped over the ice pack. Care must be taken in the application of a compression wrapping to avoid creating a tourniquet effect proximal to the area of injury. The bandages are applied in figure-of-eight fashion, avoiding circumferential wrapping as much as possible, and are removed and re-wrapped every few hours to avoid venous back-damming.

Elevation simply implies some arrangement whereby the injured part is positioned higher than the heart so that venous blood and tissue ooze gravitate away from the area of trauma. A sling is a bad device for the early treatment of a hand or wrist injury. The hurt hand is better carried cross-chest, resting on the opposite shoulder, in a Velpeau dressing when the patient is ambulatory and propped up on pillows alongside when the patient is sitting or lying down so as to place it above heart level. Extreme elevation, especially of lower extremities, may be dangerous in older patients with arterial insufficiency since it may threaten arterial flow to the part, especially when combined with compression. Such patients should be observed carefully with frequent checks of the circulation.

Cold, compression and elevation are continued until swelling has been controlled, usually two to five days. Most patients can be relied upon to carry out the mechanics of this treatment at home, once the rationale is understood by them or by some reliable family member.

If the application of local heat has any place in the treatment of acute trauma, it is after the initial period of control of bleeding and tissue ooze. It may then be cautiously started to produce some vasodilataton and hasten the absorption of the remaining exudate. Compression and intermittent elevation should be continued during the early stages of heat application until it is certain that heat is not producing more swelling.

The repair process involves the production of fibrous tissue by which the torn structures are ultimately knitted together. The healing fibrous reaction tends to be indescriminate, however, and may produce undesirable adhesion formation limiting the gliding motion of tendons, restricting the range of motion of joints, and generally causing unwanted stiffness of the injured part.

Such exercises as can be carried out without danger to the injured structures are valuable in the early stages of treatment both to prevent adhesion formation and stiffness and to hasten the absorption of the tissue exudate by the pumping action of muscular contraction. The earlier exercises can be started, the less disuse weakness and atrophy will occur and the quicker will be the rehabilitative process. Muscle strength and mass are much more easily preserved than regained. Even when rigid immobilization by splint or cast is necessary, isometric exercises of the muscles traversing the injured area can usually be carried out without harm to the damaged structures and without significant pain.

Immobilization devices should be only as large as necessary to protect the injured part and active exercises of the muscles and joints of the remainder of the extremity should be started at once. All too often, lacking specific exercise instructions, the patient with a hand injury develops stiffness of the uninjured elbow or shoulder simply by over-protecting the injured hand.

TRAUMATOLOGY OF SPECIFIC TISSUES

Certain precepts are common to the management of trauma in the various specific tissues making up the musculo-skeletal system, regardless of their anatomical location. Fractures, dislocations, sprains, strains, tendinitis, tenosynovitis and bursitis each possess generic characteristics which determine general principles of treatment. The specifics of therapy may vary with the structure and function of the anatomical region in which they lie.

Fractures

Fractures most likely to be treated in a plant dispensary are those which show little or no displacement, are inherently stable and are amenable to ambulatory treatment. Major fractures of large bones are ordinarily referred immediately to specialist care and the chief concern of the occupational physician or nurse is with adequate splinting and speedy evacuation.

Among the "minor" fractures which would seem to qualify for dispensary care are a few which, although they appear innocuous, are notorious for leading to severe degrees of disability unless specially treated. One example is a fracture at the base of the first metacarpal of the thumb. Even though the fracture fragment is small and not widely displaced, instability of the thumb carpo-metacarpal joint is likely to follow routine treatment by immobilization and the effect upon the vital post and opposition function of the thumb is ruinous. It is essential that this and similar innocent-looking but disability-threatening fractures be accurately diagnosed and identified as dangerous. Further examples of these "sleeper" fractures will be discussed in the sections dealing with each anatomical region.

Avulsion fractures is which small chips of bone are pulled off by ligaments or tendons seem minor enough and often are. Their threat lies not in the presence of the fracture but in the effect upon the stability or function of the part created by the separation of the particular ligament or tendon involved. This effect, which governs treatment, cannot be diagnosed by x-ray but demands careful clinical evaluation. Needless disability has resulted from treating the x-ray rather than the patient.

Some fractures create problems because they are not visable on x-rays made soon after the injury. Fractures heal by first mobilizing bone salts from either side of the fracture line. The fracture line is much wider ten days after fracture than it is ten minutes or ten hours post injury. Depending upon the contour of the bone, a hairline fracture may not be seen even on technically superb films until time has widened the line. Fractures of the carpal navicular bone, ribs, and insufficiency or stress fractures may all fall into this category. Injuries capable of producing such fractures must be treated as if fracture had occurred, even in the face of negative x-rays. A repeat x-ray examination ten days or two weeks later will, in most cases, deliver the final diagnosis.

Dislocations

Usually obvious and easy to diagnose, dislocations are total displacements of the opposing surfaces making up a joint. They require periods of immobilization following reduction of sufficient duration to allow complete healing of the joint capsule and supporting ligaments. Failure to carry out immobilization may mean recurrent dislocation, an especially grave threat in the shoulder. Problems arise when a simple dislocation, often of a finger, is reduced immediately by the patient or a by-stander and not reported to the examiner. Many thickened, painful, unstable finger joints have resulted from failure to recognize that a dislocation has occurred and to provide appropriate periods of support and immobilization.

Even more threatening, frequently, is the partial dislocation or subluxation in which joint surfaces have been forced apart by tearing of ligaments or the joint capsule, but frank dislocation has not occurred. Here the problem is that of determining the degree of joint instability by stress testing, comparison with the contra-lateral joint and perhaps with stress x-rays. Treatment will depend upon the degree of instability, the joint involved and the activity level of the patient. Many subluxations snap back spontaneously into normal position so there may be neither clinical nor x-ray findings of an obvious nature to alert the examiner that subluxation has occurred. Occasionally the patient will provide the clue by describing a momentary feeling of something going out of place or a deep clunk or thud as the injured part was first moved. A diagnosis of subluxation is important because it means, at very least, that a significant degree of disruption of the joint has occurred and the injury must be treated to prevent chronic joint instability.

Sprains

Sprains are defined as tearing of ligaments. Ligaments are structures designed to prevent abnormal motion of a joint while allowing normal functional motion. They are generally attached to bone above and below the joint, and forcing the joint beyond its normal range of motion will either tear the ligament fibers themselves or rip off their bony attachments, usually with a small fragment of the bone. These fractures are known as avulsion or sprain fractures and they simply provide x-ray confirmation that a significant sprain has occurred. Their treatment is the treatment of the sprain which created them.

Sprains occur in all grades of severity from the simple, mild sprain which represents the tearing of a few fibers of the ligament and does not compromise the stability of the joint to the complete tearing of the entire ligament which may leave a totally unstable joint. Between the extremes lies a whole spectrum of sprains which may be responsible for mild, moderate or severe instability of the joint. Evaluation of a sprain means accurate assessment of the degree of joint instability, for it is this feature which determines treatment. A mild sprain may need little more than symptomatic treatment and protection of the injured ligament by adhesive tape or elastic bandage for two to three weeks. Detectable joint instability of mild or moderate degree will require more rigid immobilization for up to two or three months. Total rupture of a ligament may be indication for surgical repair.

Assessment of joint instability is easiest and most likely to be accurate when performed in the early moments following injury. Having determined from examination of the opposite uninjured joint the degree of ligamentous laxity normal for the patient, the examiner then judges the amount of abnormal motion, if any, present in the injured joint. In the early examination, the point of maximum tenderness may indicate whether all or part of a ligament has been torn. If total rupture of a ligament has occurred, the gap in the ligament can sometimes be palpated at this time. Stressing the joint against the torn ligament to determine false motion or instability, while uncomfortable, is not so excruciatingly painful as to be blocked by the patient. All of these key diagnostic findings will disappear within hours as pain increases, swelling obscures the landmarks, tenderness become diffuse and muscle spasm immobilizes the part. The first examiner bears the heavy responsibility of diagnosing the degree of joint instability and, thereby, of determining treatment.

Clinical evaluation may be confirmed or refined by stress x-rays. Both the injured and the uninjured joints are x-rayed while the part is held in the position which stretches the torn ligament. The earlier such x-rays can be made after injury, the more likely they are to be meaningful. Once muscle spasm has intervened, both clinical and x-ray evaluations for joint instability may have to be done under general anaesthesia.

Failure to recognize the moderate or severe sprain with joint instability and allowing such injuries to be treated as simple sprains is almost a guarantee of significant permanent disability.

Strains

Strains are defined as tearing or severe stretching of muscle or tendon fibers. They generally result from sudden violent active contraction of the muscle rather than from the passive stress which tears or stretches ligaments and produces sprains. True strains are seen in the biceps, the hamstrings, the thigh adductors and the calf muscles most commonly, although they can occur in almost any muscle. In the true strain, there is pain on passive stretch of the involved muscle and also on active contraction of the muscle against resistance.

Muscle strain is an over-used diagnosis applied to almost any muscle which is painful. Many cases of low back pain are diagnosed as strain when, in fact, no episode capable of stretching or tearing muscle fibers has occurred. The back muscles may be painful and tender to palpation, but this generally is the result of protective muscle spasm. Usually, there is no pain when the muscle is contracted against resistance.

The common delayed muscle pain following unaccustomed activity is almost certainly not strain, by accurate definition, although it is often so diagnosed. Seldom do symptoms occur during the actual performance of the activity, and it is difficult to conceive that significant stretching or tearing of muscle fibers could occur in complete symptomatic silence. A more logical explanation is that chemical changes in the muscle due to the piling up of the metabolites of muscle contraction cause the pain. Physical conditioning, which prevents the reaction, promotes more efficient muscle metabolism and increases the blood supply to the muscle.

As is the case with sprains, strains may be mild, moderate or severe, the most severe being, of course, total rupture of the musculo-tendinous unit. Mild and moderate strains produce varying degrees of hemorrhage within the muscle and are treated by the usual routine of cold, compression and elevation until bleeding and tissue ooze is controlled. Crutches may be necessary for a time for moderate strains of calf and hamstring muscles. Wrapping the entire muscle with an elastic bandage generally makes the recovery period more comfortable. In athletes, a moderate strain of a weight bearing muscle such as a hamstring or a gastrocnemius may entail a long period of incapacity and the risk of recurrence is high.

The total rupture of a muscle or tendon must be diagnosed early since surgical repair is frequently indicated. As in the evaluation of sprains, the first examiner has the best opportunity to make an accurate assessment. The gap in the tendon is fairly easy to palpate soon after injury and the loss of power of muscle contraction is more obvious at this time. Later on, swelling may make accurate palpation impossible and substitution of intact muscles to take over the function of the torn muscle may make diagnosis difficult.

Tendinitis

Certain tendons, because of anatomical constriction or unusual functional demands, undergo attritional changes at a relatively early age and may give rise to symptoms. The minor injuries of everyday living produce microscopic tears and ravelings of the tendon fibers. Since tendons have virtually no blood supply, they are incapable of self repair and the damage becomes incremental. The accumulation of minor damage results in a roughened, nubby tendon which may produce friction and irritation of its sheath and sometimes of neighboring bursae. Ultimately the tendon may become so weakened that it ruptures.

Tendinitis is most likely to occur in tendons which operate in restricted bony channels or tunnels, such as the long head of the biceps in the bicipital groove of the upper humerus or the thumb tendons in the radial groove at the wrist, or in tendons which have to assume supportive function for a joint, such as the rotator cuff tendons of the shoulder.

Symptoms occur when, for reasons that are obscure, an inflammatory reaction begins in the damaged tendon area. The inflammatory tissue carries with it a blood supply for tendon repair, but also a nerve supply which makes for what may be extremely severe pain. Calcification of the tendon, visable by x-ray, may occur in connection with this reaction of degeneration and inflammation and the condition is then known as calcific tendinitis.

Tenosynovitis

Tendons glide within sheaths which secrete a slippery mucoid substance to act as a lubricant. Excessive repetitive motion of the tendon in its sheath, especially if the tendon excursion is long, may overwhelm the lubricating ability of the sheath and precipitate, by friction, an inflammatory reaction in the tendon sheath. This is known as tenosynovitis and is fairly common in finger and wrist tendons, some of which may have excursions of two inches or more within their sheaths. In other locations, a tendon, rough and irregular with attritional changes, may abrade the sheath and evoke an inflammatory reaction.

In its acute form, tenosynovitis responds well to short-term immobilization of the tendon and the use of anti-inflammatory drugs, such as steroid compounds, either systemically or by local injection. In the chronic form, the tendon sheath may thicken and impede the gliding motion of the tendon, sometimes actually locking the tendon so that it cannot move at all. This is seen most commonly in the flexor tendons of the fingers or thumb where it is known as trigger finger or trigger thumb. Here, anti-inflammatory treatment is less likely to be successful and it may be necessary to open up the constricted tendon sheath surgically.

Bursitis
    Bursae are anti-friction devices. Normally, a bursa is a cob-web thin sac scantily filled with a lubricating fluid similar to that found in tendon sheaths and in joints. The walls of the sac, gliding upon each other on the thin interposed layer of lubricant, dissipate friction between adjoining structures. The human body contains some two hundred bursae scattered about where bony prominences come close to the surface and may be exposed to friction from the outside or where tendons or ligaments may rub against prominences.
    When subject to unusual friction, bursae respond, at first, by oversecreting lubricating fluid and the bursal sac becomes enlarged and distended. A single blow to a bursa overlying a bony prominence, such as the tip or the elbow, may cause hemorrhage into the bursal sac. If abnormal friction persists, the walls of the sac become thickened and inflamed and the bursitis becomes chronic.
    Acute bursitis is usually treated by aspiration of the excess fluid, whether it be the normal clear lubricant or blood or a mixture of both, and injection of a steroid compound. A compression dressing is applied in an effort to prevent the re-accumulation of fluid, and the area is padded against further irritation. The more recent and the more acute is the bursitis, the more likely is this treatment to be successful. Chronically inflamed and thickened bursal sacs are less likely to respond to such treatment and may have to be surgically excised.

REGIONAL ORTHOPAEDIC PRINCIPLES

    Slightly different general principles of management apply according to whether an upper extremity or a lower extremity condition is being treated. The anatomical distribution map of orthopaedic cases (Figure 1) shows that about 42 percent of reported cases involved the upper extremity and, of these, more than three-fifths occurred in the hand. The lower extremity was affected in about 29 percent of on-the-job injuries or work-related conditions.

Upper Extremity

The upper extremity can be viewed as a complex articulated device designed to place the hand in optimal position for function. Pain or loss of motion in the shoulder, elbow or wrist causes disability chiefly because of inability properly to position the hand. The key principle in the management of upper extremity conditions is to preserve mobility at almost any cost.

To this end, fractures are immobilized for the minimum time necessary for satisfactory healing, and many are not immobilized at all. When there must be rigid fixation, the immobilizing device is rigged so as to interfere as little as possible with the mobility of the rest of the extremity. Swelling is vigorously combatted because it leads to stiffness. Exercise of all uninjured joints in the extremity is begun on the first day of treatment and rigorously supervised throughout. Where fractures are impacted or inherently stable and displacement or angulation is not too severe, it may be elected to accept minor architectural abnormality in favor of retained mobility and such injuries may be protected only for the few days of acute discomfort.

A major exception to the rule of playing for mobility in the care of upper extremity conditions occurs in certain injuries of the thumb, especially those affecting the carpo-metacarpal and the metacarpo-phlangeal joints. Here, although mobility is important to allow approximation of the thumb to all fingers, stability is even more vital if the thumb is to fulfill its function as post and opposer to the fingers in grasp and pinch. It may also become necessary at times, especially in conditions of the wrist, to trade some motion for relief of pain if the pain is so severe as seriously to hamper hand function.

In the diagnosis of the more obscure conditions of the upper extremity, the possibility of referred pain should be kept in mind. The nerve supply of the arm derives from nerve roots which exit the spinal canal between the lower cervical vertebrae, and it is never amiss to evaluate the neck when baffling symptoms present in the upper extremity, especially in the shoulder area. The ability to reproduce the atypical pain of a shoulder complaint by laterally flexing the neck toward the painful side and then pushing down sharply on the head may quickly exonerate the shoulder from responsibility for the complaint and correctly direct attention to the cervical spine.

In another extremely common referral phenomenon, pain originating in the shoulder may be felt at the point of insertion of the deltoid muscle, halfway down the upper arm, and there often is impressive local tenderness at this point. The patient may even protest examination of the shoulder for complaints that seem to center at a much lower point.

Lower Extremity

In the lower extremity, stability and painless weight bearing are the primary goals and, if necessary, some mobility may be traded for stability. Fractures involving joint surfaces must be meticulously reduced so as to restore smooth articulating surfaces, by open reduction if necessary. Otherwise, the high compression stress of weight bearing will produce pain and disability as the changes of traumatic arthritis occur. Fractures are rigidily immobilized for long periods until it is absolutely certain that healing is complete and full stability has been achieved.

Ligamentous injuries which threaten the stability of weight bearing joints must be identified early and treated aggressively with long periods of immobilization or, occasionally, open repair of the ligament to avoid lax, unreliable joints. Unstable joints not only predispose to recurrent injury, but they, too, degenerate into traumatic arthritis and become chronically painful and disabling.

Early exercise is as important in the lower extremity as it is in the upper, but for different reasons. Joints of the lower extremity, especially the knee, depend upon muscle power for stability. Exercises are aimed at the preservation of muscle power and mass. An architecturally perfect knee with smooth articulating surfaces and intact ligaments can become unstable, painful and disabling if weakness of the quadriceps and hamstring muscles is allowed to occur and persist.

Referred pain in the lower extremity is common because of the high incidence of low back conditions which involve the lower lumbar and upper sacral nerve roots. These pain patterns are generally better known and more easily recognized than those in the upper extremity.

The pain of vascular insufficiency (intermittent claudication), is often confused with musculo-skeletal pain. Checking the pedal, popliteal and femoral pulses is a useful part of the orthopaedic evaluation of lower extremity complaints.

The common referral of pain originating in the hip to the knee is worth bearing in mind. The patient with knee complaints unsubstantiated by clear-cut local findings has not been adequately examined until the hip has also been thoroughly evaluated.

CHAPTER 2
THE HAND (253)

Combining the most delicate tactile sensitivity with the capacity for precisely integrated motion as well as for powerful pinch and grasp, the hand is truly the design masterpiece of the musculo-skeletal system. Intricacy of design and diversity of function, however, impose special burdens upon the management of hand injuries. Stiffness from post traumatic adhesion formation and immobilization develops quickly, and even minor disruption of the complex structure of the hand can lead to high degree of functional impairment.

As in all anatomical areas, structure and function combine to determine the vulnerability of the part both to acute injury and to long term attritional changes. Long, lightly-boned, multi-jointed, highly mobile fingers, nearly devoid of muscle support, forecast a high incidence of fractures, sprains and dislocations.

The major muscles responsible for finger and thumb motion lie in the forearm and transmit their power by long tendons gliding within lengthy tendon sheaths. The tendon excursion necessary to flex the middle finger fully into the palm is more than two inches. Moreover, the capability of the tendons to produce varying degrees of flexion and extension of each of the three joints of the fingers independent of the others entails complex mechanisms with sliding clutches, tethering devices and pulleys. Conditions are obviously ideal for the development of tenosynovitis.

It is not surprising that the most frequent orthopaedic hand problems are fractures (208), sprains (18), dislocations (10) and tenosynovitis (11). Hand lacerations, including those of tendons, are not included in the 1,000 case sample of orthopaedic conditions. By local usage, major hand and tendon lacerations are referred to hand surgeons for treatment.

For purposes of medical record keeping and legal reporting, clear anatomical designation of injuries and defects is important. The terminology suggested in Figure 2 is generally accepted and avoids the confusion of numbering the fingers.

25

Before considering individual diagnostic entities, some general suggestions for the treatment of all hand injuries are listed in Table 2.

1. Remove finger rings before swelling develops.

2. Immobilize only those joints necessary for healing of the injury and preserve function in all others from the first day of treatment.

3. Arrange immobilization devices to interfere as little as possible with overall hand function. Ring and little fingers, for instance, move together and may be splinted together as a unit when either is injured. This often allows better function than when either is splinted separately.

4. Immobilize only as long as necessary for healing. Often the period of rigid fixation can be shortened and an injured finger mobilized safely by strapping it to an adjacent finger for support. Use the functional units (ring and little, index and middle).

5. Treat injuries which threaten the stability of the thumb with special care. Loss of the post and opposition function of the thumb because of painful instability is a disaster to hand function.

6. Give specific instructions for regular exercises of the proximal upper extremity joints. A stiff elbow or shoulder is a high price to pay for the treatment of an injured hand.

Table 2. General suggestions for the treatment of all hand injuries.

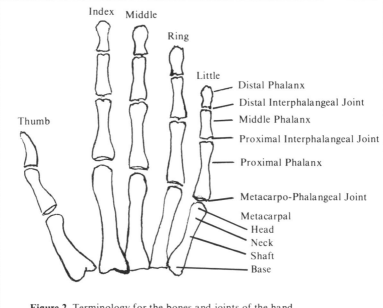

Figure 2. Terminology for the bones and joints of the hand.

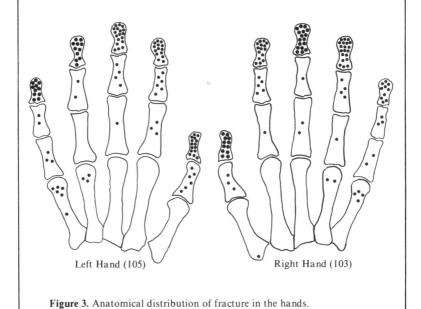

Left Hand (105)   Right Hand (103)

Figure 3. Anatomical distribution of fracture in the hands.

FRACTURES (208)

Figure 3 is a map showing the anatomical distribution of fractures in the hands. Fractures account for more than 80 percent of all hand injuries, and nearly three-quarters of all hand fractures occur in the distal phalanges.

Distal Phalanx (152)

Distal phalanx fractures account for 60 percent of all hand injuries. Most result from a severe pinch or crush of the finger tip and involve shattering or comminution of the spongy vascular bone of the distal tuft of the phalanx without much displacement (Figure 4). Most heal quickly without any need for special splinting, although a padded finger cap for a week or two affords comfort and protection during the healing period. The patient is more likely to use the hand normally if the injured finger tip is protected from the inevitable bumping and irritation of daily use.

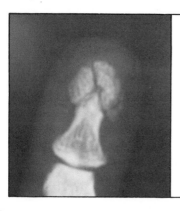

Figure 4. Fracture of the distal phalanx of a finger with comminution of the spongy bone of the tuft.

The distal phalangeal compartment behaves like a closed space, sealed off from the remainder of the finger by a water-tight bulkhead. Hemorrhage into this space from the crushed bone and tissue causes an increase in pressure and produces severe pain. Unless the space has been opened by compounding of the fracture, it is often necessary to vent the compartment by drilling a hole near the base of the fingernail. A bluish half-moon of discoloration under the nail indicates both the need for and the site of drilling. The nail may be punctured by gently twirling the sharp tip of a knife blade after careful cleansing of the site and the patient may well be spared a sleepless night.

About one-fifth of distal phalanx fractures are compound, usually from within due to bursting of the skin by the crush. These require careful wound cleansing and close observation since infection can develop easily in the crushed and devitalized tissues. Prophylactic antibiotics are sometimes used in particularly dirty injuries. The risk of infection is even higher in those that are compounded by penetration from without, the degree of danger depending upon the nature of the penetrating object and the possibility that foreign material may have been punched into the depths of the wound. Surgical exploration of the wound and debridement may be necessary.

Avulsion fracture of the extensor tendon (9) is a different type of distal phalanx fracture which deserves special comment. The injury results from sudden forced flexion of the extended distal phalanx, as when a ball strikes the end of the finger. The bony insertion of the extensor tendon is torn from the base of the phalanx (Figure 5). Usually, the avulsed fragment of bone is small and not widely displaced. Occasionally, the tendon pulls away from the bone without creating an avulsion chip, so the x-ray cannot be counted upon to make the diagnosis in all cases. In any event, the patient loses the ability actively to extend the distal phalanx. The injury is commonly called baseball finger or drop finger.

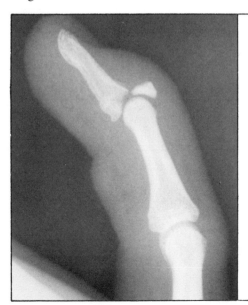

Figure 5. Typical avulsion fracture of the insertion of the extensor tendon into the base of the distal phalanx.

Most such injuries can be treated with a full length finger splint holding the distal phalanx in a position of maximum hyper-extension, the degree of hyper-extension being determined by that present in the opposite normal finger. Fixation must be consistently maintained for six to eight weeks. Care must be taken to pad the strapping across the top of the distal interphalangeal joint since it is mainly the pressure of this strap which maintains the hyper-extended position. The splint extends to the base of the finger and metacarpo-phalangeal joint motion is permitted.

If the avulsion fracture fragment is large, involving more than 25 percent of the joint surface, or widely displaced, the patient should be referred for specialist care since open reduction and internal fixation will probably be necessary.

Patients with extensor tendon avulsions occasionally report late and the question arises as to how long after injury closed treatment can successfully be used. Excellent results have beenreported by splinting initiated up to three weeks following injury in patients who, if seen immediately, would qualify for this form of treatment. It is probably worthwhile to proceed with closed treatment within this time span. Beyond three weeks following injury and in cases where splinting has not been consistently maintained throughout the six to eight week period, surgical reattachment of the tendon may be indicated. Some permanent loss of the flexion range of the distal interphalangeal joint frequently follows surgical treatment.

Middle Phalanx (27) and Proximal Phalanx (23)

Fractures of the middle phalanx and of the proximal phalanx may be considered together from the standpoint of treatment. In both, angulation, if it occurs, will usually be palmar in direction and is due to the pull of the intrinsic muscles of the hand which insert on the flexor surfaces of the phalanges. Figure 6A and B shows the typical palmar angulation of a fracture of the proximal phalanx of the middle finger as seen in lateral and oblique views. This angulation can frequently be reduced simply by placing the finger in a position of flexion so as to relax the pull of the intrinsic muscles. Figure 6C shows the result of this maneuver as applied to the fracture seen in Figure 6A and B. If acceptable position is achieved, the finger is splinted in a position of flexion (50 to 60 degrees at both the metacarpo-phalangeal joint and the proximal interphalangeal joint). For stability, a full length splint extending well up the forearm is necessary. One convenient method for

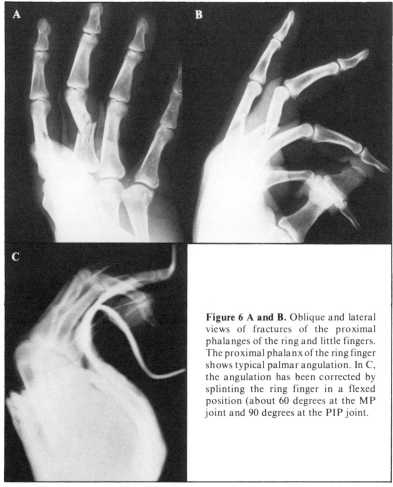

Figure 6 A and B. Oblique and lateral views of fractures of the proximal phalanges of the ring and little fingers. The proximal phalanx of the ring finger shows typical palmar angulation. In C, the angulation has been corrected by splinting the ring finger in a flexed position (about 60 degrees at the MP joint and 90 degrees at the PIP joint.

the immobilization of proximal and middle phalanx fractures is to embed a long aluminum finger splint in a plaster forearm cast. Once the plaster has set, the splint can be bent to any desired angle. Extreme care must be taken in positioning the splinted finger to avoid rotational deformity. When flexed, all fingers point toward the scaphoid tubercle on the radial side of the palmar aspect of the wrist. Check the flexed position of the opposite normal finger and be certain that the splinted position of the injured finger matches.

The usual immobilization time for shaft fractures of the proximal and middle phalanges is about three weeks. A further period of partial immobilization and protection by strapping to an adjacent uninjured finger as outlined under general suggestions for treatment is often useful.

If fractures are oblique, unstable, severely comminuted or overriding, expert care is necessary and traction or open reduction may be required. Even seemingly stable fractures should be checked by x-ray after 48 hours of immobilization to be sure they have not angulated or displaced.

Avulsion fracture of the volar plate (*) is a special fracture of the palmar aspect of the base of the middle phalanx. It is not represented in this sampling of cases, but deserves special comment. Usually the result of a hyper-extension injury of the proximal interphalangeal joint, a small triangle of bone is avulsed from the base of the middle phalanx. Although innocent in appearance (Figure 7), this fracture signals significant disruption of the joint and subluxation is very likely to occur. Any such fracture which involves more than 15 percent of the joint surface should be referred for specialist care and will probably require open reduction and internal fixation. Smaller avulsions may be treated by splinting in flexion, but should be followed closely by x-ray

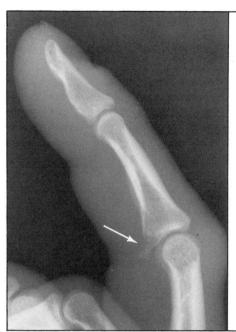

Figure 7. A notorious "sleeper" fracture which appears insignificant and is often hard to see. The avulsed bony fragment from the base of the middle phalanx threatens subluxation and permanent instability of the proximal interphalangeal joint.

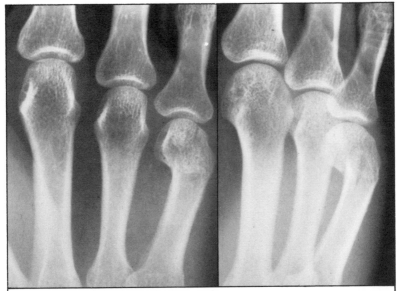

Figure 8. Fracture of the neck of the fifth metacarpal caused by impact upon the fist. The head fragment is angulated about 45 degrees into the palm.

to detect subluxation.

Metacarpal (16)

Most commonly injured are the necks of the ring and little finger metacarpals, usually by direct impact upon the clenched or fisted hand. The head of the metacarpal is angulated into the palm and, generally, firmly impacted (Figure 8).

In the interests of the preservation of mobility, angulation of the head fragment of less than 45 degrees is usually accepted and no reduction is undertaken. A full length finger splint extending above the wrist is applied, largely for comfort, since the fracture is quite stable. After a week or two, the splint can generally be removed and the finger mobilized with adhesive or elastic bandage support. Although fracture healing time is about six weeks, the patient is generally comfortable and using the hand normally before this time. There may be a slight cosmetic defect due to loss of the knuckle prominence.

When the head fragment is angulated more than 45 degrees, referral should be made for consideration of reduction. Closed reduction of these fractures usually requires general anaesthesia, forceful mani-

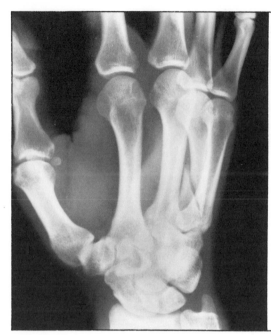

Figure 9. Fracture of the shaft of the fourth metacarpal. Even though oblique and slightly over-riding, this fracture is likely to be stable because of splinting by adjacent intact metacarpals.

pulation to break up the impaction, and post-reduction immobilization in a position of full flexion of the finger for several weeks. The functional loss due to the rigors of treatment may be significant, and it is for this reason that lesser degrees of angulation of the head fragment are accepted and the finger mobilized as rapidly as tolerated.

Fractures of the shafts of the finger metacarpals (Figure 9), although often oblique, are usually quite stable because of the neighboring intact metacarpals and the fact that the metacarpals are snugly bound together by soft tissues. An elastic bandage wrap of the hand is frequently sufficient support. Heavy use of the hand should, of course, be interdicted for the three to four week period of symptoms.

Fracture of the base of the thumb metacarpal (1) is a fracture - dislocation of the carpo-metacarpal joint and almost always requires open reduction and internal fixation. The articular surface of the carpal bone at the base of the thumb is saddle-shaped and the base of the thumb metacarpal fits into the saddle as do the buttocks of a rider. The fracture (Figure 10) usually splits off one buttock and dislocates the other buttock along with the remainder of the metacarpal. The architecture and stability of the joint is destroyed.

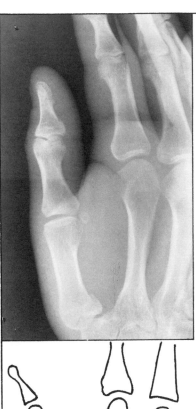

Figure 10. The x-ray shows a typical fracture through the base of the thumb metacarpal. Drawing A demonstrates the position of the fracture line and Drawing B indicates the potential for displacement with dislocation of the carpo-metacarpal joint and total loss of stability of the thumb.

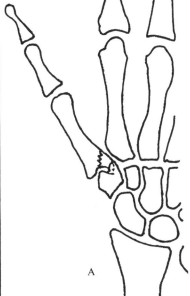

A

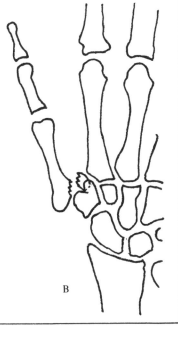

B

Loss of motion and stability of the thumb carpo-metacarpal joint compromises the post and opposition function of the thumb and this, in turn, severely impairs the function of the entire hand.

SPRAINS (18)

Proximal interphalangeal joint sprains (13) usually involve the lateral ligaments of the joints and result from an impacting type of injury on the extended finger which forces it out of line. They may be associated with tiny avulsion chip fractures. They are notoriously refractory to treatment and frequently produce permanent partial disability with thickening of the joint and partial loss of motion.

Various methods of treating these injuries have been tried, including prolonged immobilization, early mobilization, intensive physiotherapy, and even local injection with steroid drugs, all without signal success. Probably the best of a dubious lot of treatments is immobilization on a finger splint in a position of slight flexion for two to three weeks, followed by protected mobilization with the injured finger strapped to the next normal finger until reasonably comfortable. The patient should be warned at the outset of the probability of a protracted course and the possibility of mild permanency.

Sprain of the metacarpo-phalangeal joint of the thumb (5) (game-keeper's thumb, ski-pole thumb) is always a potentially serious injury because the stability of the joint is threatened and, with it, efficient post and opposition function of the thumb. The degree of lateral instability of the joint must be carefully determined, using the same joint of the opposite thumb as the standard.

Mild or moderate instability with stress pain, usually of the ulnar side ligament, is treated by rigid splinting of the thumb in the position of slight flexion which the normal relaxed thumb assumes on a full length splint extending to wrist level for a period of three to six weeks, depending on the degree of instability. On removal of the splint, the thumb is protected by a firm basket-weave adhesive strapping of the metacarpo-phalangeal joint for another two to three weeks. Support with an elastic bandage figure-of-eight wrapping is provided for rugged work or athletic activity until the thumb is painless on full normal function.

Severe lateral instability requires specialist consultation for consideration of open repair of the ligament in the fresh injury or of arthrodesis of the joint in old or neglected injuries with significant pain and disability.

As in proximal interphalangeal joint sprains, there may be avulsion fractures, but these only confirm, by x-ray, the presence of ligamentous injury and do not influence treatment unless they are very large and widely displaced, in which case open reduction and internal fixation may be indicated.

DISLOCATIONS (10)

Dislocations usually involve the **distal interphalangeal joints (5)** or the **proximal interphalangeal joints (3)** of the fingers. The more distal bone of the joint is usually dislocated dorsally (Figure 11). If seen shortly after injury, they can usually be reduced without anaesthesia by simple traction on the finger accompanied by downward pressure on the dorsally displaced base of the phalanx. Following reduction, they should by splinted in a position of mild flexion for three weeks. Protective strapping to the next finger during the ensuing mobilization period is then used until joint swelling has disappeared and the finger is comfortable.

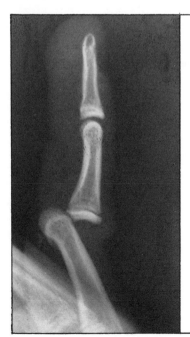

Figure 11. Typical dislocation of the proximal interphalangeal joint of a finger. Such dislocations are usually easily reduced but must be rigidly splinted to allow stable healing of the supportive structures of the joint.

Many of these dislocations will be reduced by fellow workers, teammates, or the patient at the site of the accident and may arrive at the dispensary already reduced and quite comfortable. It is important to proceed with immobilization as outlined above, however, to avoid a permanently unstable and painful joint.

Metacarpo-phalangeal joint dislocations (2) often cannot be reduced by closed manipulation because of interposition of soft tissue between the joint surfaces. If one attempt at reduction by traction and pressure on the dislocated bone is unsuccessful, the patient should be referred promptly for open reduction.

TENOSYNOVITIS (11)

Acute tenosynovitis (7), while slightly more common in the flexors, may involve either the flexor or extensor tendons of the fingers. It usually follows some unaccustomed highly repetitive activity. All of the clinical signs of inflammation including swelling, redness and increased local heat are present and, in addition, there may be palpable or even audible creaking or crepitus on motion of the involved tendon in its sheath.

Response to treatment by immobilization of the involved finger and systemic steroids is usually prompt. If there is no medical contra-indication, steroids are givin in full therapeutic dosage for three days, in declining dosage for four days, and discontinued at the end of a week. If the use of systemic sterioid drugs is contra-indicated, it is possible to inject local steroids into the point of maximum tenderness in the tendon or tendon sheath. There is, however, at least a statistical chance of tendon rupture following the local injection of steroids.

Because of the element of individual susceptibility to tenosynovitis, the danger of recurrence is real, and attempts should be made to protect the patient from highly repetitive work in the future.

Chronic stenosing tenosynovitis (4) involves thickening of the tendon sheath to the point that the normal smooth gliding motion of the tendon is impeded. In the hand, this usually occurs in the finger or thumb flexors at the level of the palmar creases and presents as trigger finger (1) or trigger thumb (1). Ordinarily, there is no clear history of past bouts of acute tenosynovitis, but the patient may have noted soreness in the tendon area for several weeks prior to the onset of triggering. In true triggering, the patient is able actively to flex the finger or thumb normally, but is unable to extend it, and must reach over with the other hand and peel the affected finger or thumb back into the extended position. There is an instant of pain and sometimes an audible snap as the tendon is pulled through the stenosed segment of the sheath.

Involvement of the long abductor and short extensor tendons of the thumb where they lie in a deep groove in the distal radius is known as de Quervain's disease (2) and, while technically a condition of the wrist, manifests itself as pain on attempt to move the thumb away from the remainder of the hand. The patient is unable to bridge a wide span and may also have difficulty with activities requiring a combination of firm grip and forearm roll, as in wringing out a washcloth.

Treatment of chronic stenosing tenosynovitis by local injection of steroids is occasionally successful. Surgical incision of the thickened and stenosed portion of the tendon sheath is usually necessary and is generally simple and satisfactory.

CONTUSIONS AND CRUSH INJURIES (6)

The severely contused or crushed hand requires careful attention and close follow-up despite the fact that a negative x-ray may lull the examiner into the assumption that the injury is trivial. Post traumatic effusion may become very extensive and diffuse and the resultant adhesion formation may have a ruinous effect upon the highly integrated function of the hand.

If the blow is to the dorsum of the hand, the extensor tendons may be impacted against the metacarpal bones and acute tenosynovitis may develop. Contusions of the palm may result in severe bleeding and effusion beneath the firm and unyielding palmar aponeurosis with acute pain and, occasionally, pressure interference with circulation to the fingers. Contusions of the heel of the hand may damage the intrinsic muscles of the thumb and little finger and produce long periods of pain and disability.

In all hand contusions and crush injuries, compression bandages should be carefully applied, ideally over sheet wadding, mechanic's waste or other padding material after the initial use of ice packs. The hand should be elevated and forced active exercises of the fingers and thumb begun immediately. The patient with a crushed hand should be seen daily for observation, re-arrangement of compression bandages and reinforcement of the exercise routine. Formal physiotherapy may be extremely helpful, once the tissue ooze has been brought under control.

CHAPTER 3
THE WRIST (68)

The wrist, in addition to the joints between the eight small carpal bones, includes the joint between the distal radius and ulna, the joints joining the two forearm bones to the carpal complex, and the joints between the carpal bones and the bases of the metacarpals (Figure 12). This multiplicity of joints allows fine tuning of hand position, once approximate placement has been accomplished by the shoulder and the elbow.

The wrist is capable of hinge motion of 60 to 90 degrees in each direction (dorsi-flexion and palmar-flexion) and of side-to-side motion of 15 to 30 degrees toward either the little finger (ulnar deviation) or the thumb (radial deviation). These ranges not only place the hand in optimal position for function but also properly tension the muscles for

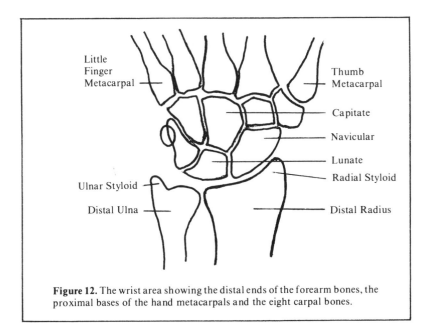

Figure 12. The wrist area showing the distal ends of the forearm bones, the proximal bases of the hand metacarpals and the eight carpal bones.

the task at hand. Maximum power grip, for instance, is achieved with the wrist in about 30 degrees of dorsiflexion. In this position, the finger and thumb flexors are at the proper length to deliver maximum power. The wrist also shares the important motion of forearm roll with the elbow. The range from the palm-down position of pronation to the palm-up position of supination is achieved by rotation of the distal radius through an arc of 180 degrees about the distal ulna at the radio-ulnar joint.

The wrist is a conduit through which pass the major tendons of the hand and all of its blood and nerve supply. Some of the structural arrangements for the passage of this multiplex of tissues through the narrow isthmus of the wrist create clinical problems.

On the palm side of the wrist, the contour of the carpal bones and a bridging ligament form a tunnel within which lie the flexor tendons and the median nerve. Swelling of the carpal joints or of any of the contents of this rigid tunnel may lead to pressure upon the median nerve and produce carpal tunnel syndrome, a fairly common cause of symptoms.

On the radial side of the wrist, two thumb tendons pass through a bony groove in the distal radius which is also converted into a tunnel by a roofing ligament. Highly repetitive thumb motion may lead to inflammation and thickening of the sheaths of these tendons, interfering with the normal gliding motion, and resulting in pain and restriction of thumb motion (de Quervain's disease).

On the dorsal side of the wrist, a pulley arrangement abruptly alters the direction of pull of another thumb tendon responsible for dorsally cocking the thumb. Friction at this pulley occasionally produces tendinitis and even rupture of this tendon. Moreover, the thumb extensor tendon angles sharply across two of the extensor tendons of the wrist and may, by friction, create inflammatory irritation in them. This condition is known as cross-over tendinitis.

Quite apart from the characteristics of structure and function incidental to normal use, the wrist is peculiarly vulnerable to injury in falls because of the reflex protective mechanism which almost automatically thrusts the arm out as a shock-absorber strut to cushion body impact. The shock wave is transmitted upward from the heel of the hand along the radial side of the wrist and then up the forearm to the elbow. Given sufficient force, fracture somewhere along this line of transmission frequently occurs. At wrist level, either the carpal navicular or the distal end of the radius will be the likely victims.

The peculiarities of structure and the demands of both normal and emergency function suggest vulnerability of the wrist to fractures (26) and to tenosynovitis (19). The multiplicity of joints and tendons make the wrist a prime site for ganglion (10), a cyst-like mass which usually arises from joint capsules or tendon sheaths.

FRACTURES (26)

Carpal Navicular (7)

The carpal navicular, second largest of the eight carpal bones, lies along the thumb side of the wrist directly in the line of transmitted force in a fall on the outstretched hand. In such a fall, it is pinioned between two lesser carpal bones which lie at the base of the thumb and the wedge-shaped styloid process of the radius. The navicular usually fractures across its narrow waist as the upward force rams it against the anvil of the radial styloid.

Because of its peculiar shape and position, fractures of the carpal navicular are notoriously difficult to visualize by x-ray immediately following injury. They are seldom significantly displaced and the fracture line usually lies in a plane which is not parallel with the beam of the x-ray in routine positioning of the wrist for x-ray examination.

A special carpal navicular view (Figure 13) gives optimal x-ray visualization of the area and should always be ordered if fracture is suspected. This is a modified antero-posterior view with the wrist positioned, palm down, on the film holder and the x-ray tube directed vertically downward. In this special technique, the wrist and film holder are mounted on an inclined plane of 10 degrees from the horizontal with the hand higher than the elbow. The hand is angled toward the little finger side so the thumb becomes an extension of the forearm. This position throws the navicular into contour and exposes the waist area of the bone where fractures are most likely to occur.

Figure 14 demonstrates the efficacy of the special carpal navicular view. It shows three x-ray views of an injured wrist made shortly after injury. Figure 14A, a routine antero-posterior view, is not diagnostic for fracture. The small arrow on the film indicates the narrow waist of the bone where fracture has occurred. Figure 14B is a routine oblique view which, with the aid of the arrow, is somewhat more suspicious for fracture, but not diagnositc. Figure 14C is the special carpal navicular view and quite clearly shows the fracture line across the waist of the bone.

Even this special technique may fail to reveal a fracture line in the

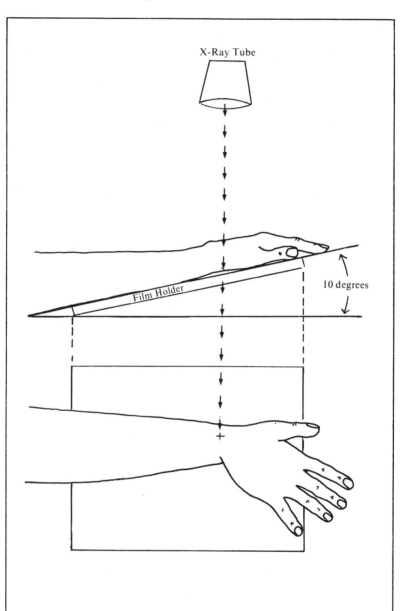

X-Ray Tube

Film Holder

10 degrees

Figure 13. Special carpal navicular x-ray of the wrist. An antero-posterior view with the forearm, wrist and hand angled upward 10 degrees and the hand placed in ulnar deviation so the thumb becomes an extension of the long axis of the forearm. The x-ray beam is directed vertically.

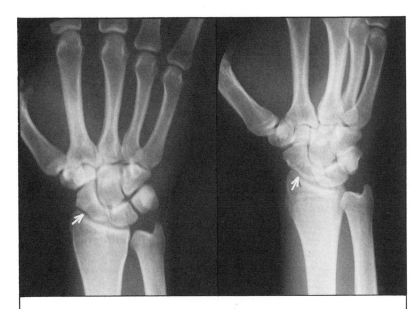

Figure 14. Routine antero-posterior and oblique views of an injured wrist are not clearly diagnostic of fracture of the navicular. Arrows indicate position of fracture line. X-ray below of the same wrist made at the same time, but by the technique shown in Figure 13, clearly delineates the fracture across the waist of the carpal navicular.

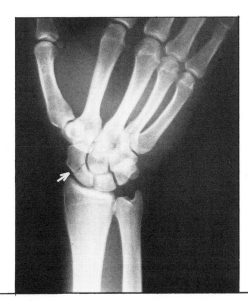

fresh injury, however, and it may be necessary to wait for ten days or two weeks and repeat the x-ray examination to diagnose or exclude fracture. During this time interval, the fracture line, if present, will become wider and more clearly visable by x-ray because of the normal absorption of bone from either side of the fracture line which occurs early in the process of healing.

The rule, then, is to treat every injured wrist presenting with a history and findings consistent with carpal navicular fracture as if it were fractured, regardless of the initial x-ray findings. A history of a fall, landing on the outstretched hand, followed by pain in the wrist with local tenderness in the dimpled area on the radial side of the wrist between the base of the thumb and the tip of the radial styloid is sufficient evidence upon which to initiate rigid casting or splinting of the wrist exactly as would be done were carpal navicular fracture diagnosed. If a repeated x-ray examination, including the special carpal navicular view, two weeks later fails to reveal any fracture, rigid fixation may be discontinued and the wrist mobilized with an elastic bandage support. The diagnosis then becomes sprain of the wrist, but it should be noted that this is a diagnosis of exclusion, and is almost never made immediately following injury.

Because of poor blood supply, fractures of the carpal navicular heal slowly and aseptic necrosis of one fragment is fairly common. Cast fixation will be necessary for a minimum of 10 to 12 weeks and, in many cases, for an even longer period. The first cast usually extends above the elbow, maintaining the forearm in thumb-up or mid-position between pronation and supination, the wrist in mild dorsi-flexion and radial deviation, and includes the thumb. After six weeks, this can be changed to a forearm cast which includes the metacarpo-phalangeal joint of the thumb, but leaves the interphalangeal joint free.

Cast maintenance becomes a problem since the patient is usually free of pain after the first two or three weeks and may use the casted hand vigorously, often softening the palm portion by exposure to water and the pressure of tool handles and the like. Continued rigid fixation throughout the healing period is important, and frequent cast changes and repairs may be necessary to maintain adequate immobilization.

Failure to achieve bony union of carpal navicular fractures can ususally be attributed either to lack of early immobilization because of difficulty in identifying the fracture, or to lapses in rigid fixation because of cast break-down.

If there is failure of primary treatment manifested either by non-union or by avascular necrosis of one fragment, the patient should be referred for specialist opinion and treatment. A variety of open procedures are available depending upon the condition of the wrist and the functional demands of the patient. Established non-union or aseptic necrosis almost invariably spells significant permanent disability.

Distal Radius (17)

If the carpal navicular escapes, the next point of severe impact in a fall on the outstretched hand is the expanded end of the distal radius. The upward thrust shatters the end of the radius, pushing it upward toward the forearm and tilting its joint surface toward the dorsal surface of the wrist (Figure 15). This is the classical Colles fracture (15). When severely comminuted and displaced, reduction under general anaesthesia will usually be necessary. Occasionally, the severity of comminution makes retention of closed reduction impossible and skeletal traction or internal fixation must be used. Patients with severe Colles fractures are simply splinted and referred for specialist care in most instances.

Cast fixation is usually required for six to eight weeks and, in order to hold the jumble of comminuted fragments in satisfactory position, it is often necessary to fix the wrist in a position of palmar flexion and ulnar

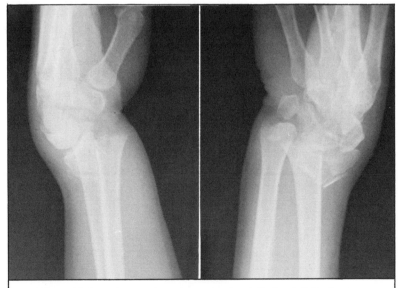

Figure 15. Severely comminuted, angulated and displaced Colles fracture seen in lateral and antero-posterior views.

deviation. This position makes use, or even exercise, of the hand difficult and this, combined with stiffness of the wrist and sometimes of the elbow and shoulder, may make rehabilitation long and discouraging.

Undisplaced or mildly displaced fractures of the distal radius (2) may be treated in short arm casts without reduction and usually heal within four to six weeks. Finger, elbow and shoulder exercises must be taught and supervised throughout the healing period.

It may be difficult to judge the degree of displacement since many of these fractures are impacted and fracture lines are sometimes not clearly visable by x-ray. It is valuable to bear the normal anatomical relationships of the wrist in mind. In the antero-posterior x-ray view, the tip of the radial styloid normally lies one centimeter distal to the tip of the ulnar styloid. In the lateral view, the articular surface of the distal radius is tilted 15 degrees toward the palm. These standards may also be useful in judging the reduction obtained in patients treated in outside medical facilities and in forming some estimate as to the probable duration and degree of disability.

Other Carpal Bone Fractures (2)

X-ray of the injured wrist may show, in the lateral view, a small bony fragment lying just dorsal to the carpal bones. The fracture can seldom be seen in the antero-posterior view and it is often impossible to determine which carpal bone has been fractured. These are often chip fractures of the large capitate bone which lies just proximal to the base of the middle finger metacarpal and result from dorsi-flexion injury of the wrist.

They can usually be treated symptomatically with a splint or half cast to the wrist for about three weeks. They generally become asymptomatic and present no disability problem although they may not heal by bony union.

DISLOCATIONS (*)

Dislocations of the wrist are not common. They are difficult to diagnose and treat. The x-ray is often confusing, and it is always appropriate to order comparable views of the opposite uninjured wrist. **Dislocation of the carpal lunate (*),** although not represented in this sampling of cases, is most likely to be encountered and is important to recognize and treat early. It usually results from a severe dorsi-flexion injury. Examination reveals a thickened, swollen and very painful wrist.

If seen immediately after injury, it may be possible to feel an abnormal bony prominence in the center of the palmar aspect of the wrist.

The carpal lunate bone, seen in the lateral view x-ray, is shaped like a quarter moon. Its concave surface holds the convexity of the capitate bone which lies between it and the bases of the metacarpals. Its convex surface fits into the concavity of the distal radius. In the antero-posterior x-ray, it lies just to the ulnar side of the navicular.

When the wrist is forced into extreme dorsi-flexion and impacted, the lunate may be popped out onto the palmar side of the wrist like a seed out of an orange. The lateral view x-ray (Figure 16A) will show the lunate quite clearly, tilted out of position toward the palm, its concave surface empty of any articulation. In the antero-posterior view (Figure 16B), the joint space between the navicular and the lunate is widened and distorted. Figures 16C and 16D show the normal position and relationships of the lunate after the dislocation has been reduced.

If seen soon after injury, the dislocation can sometimes be reduced without anaesthesia by strong traction on the hand, full dorsi-flexion of the wrist to open the space, firm finger pressure on the lunate to force it back into the carpus, and then return of the wrist to neutral or a slightly palmar-flexed position. The chance for a relatively easy reduction disappears within an hour or so as swelling obscures bony landmarks and muscle spasm locks the wrist in place. If one trial at reduction soon after injury fails, the wrist should be splinted and the patient referred for specialist care. Open reduction is often necessary.

TENOSYNOVITIS (19)

Acute tenosynovitis (14) is similar to that seen in the hand and may involve either the flexor or the extensor tendons of the wrist. It is often related to unaccustomed repetitive activity as in the hand, but may also result from activity requiring strong grip, as on the handle of a tool, plus repeated impact. Use of a pick-axe on frozen ground, for instance, or the weekend gardener's workout with hand hedge trimmers may precipitate the condition. Patients show severe pain, swelling, redness and increased local heat over the involved tendons, and the peculiar crepitus associated with tendon motion within the inflamed sheath may be detectable. Treatment is identical to that of the condition in the hand with splint immobilization and short term use of systemic steroids.

Cross-over tendinitis (5) is considered a form of tenosynovitis although the pathological details of this condition are not entirely clear. The two

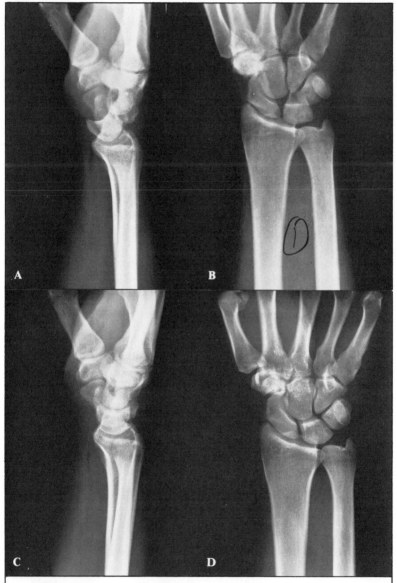

Figure 16, A and B. Lateral and antero-posterior x-rays of the wrist showing dislocation of the carpal semilunar bone. The semilunar is tilted toward the palm and its concave surface is empty. In the antero-posterior view, the space between the semilunar and the navicular is widened. Compare with post-reduction views of the same wrist (C and D).

extensor tendons of the wrist on the dorsal radial side which are over-passed by the long thumb extensor are involved. It is presumed that heavy or highly repetitive use of these muscles beneath the constricting band of the crossing thumb extensor tendon produces friction, irritation and inflammation.

Patients show swelling and tenderness on the radial side of the dorsal surface of the forearm just above the wrist. Redness and increased local heat are usually not impressive and there seldom is any tendon crepitus. Swelling and tenderness with pain on use may persist for several weeks and anti-inflammatory treatment is usually not dramatically effective. Splinting or elastic support of the tender area along with physiotherapy are generally used and a job change may be necessary.

SPRAINS (7)
Usually diagnosed by exclusion only after interval x-rays have been negative for carpal navicular fracture, wrist sprains have, for the most part, already been treated by two weeks of immobilization by the time they are diagnosed. The rigid splinting is removed and the wrist is gradually mobilized with an elastic bandage support over a further period of a week or ten days. Prognosis is good and there is no great threat of permanency.

GANGLION (10)
Ganglions are cysts filled with a thick, glairy, gel-like substance. They usually communicate with joints or with tendon sheaths and their content is probably the normal lubricating fluid of joints and tendon sheaths, concentrated and partially inspissated by seclusion within the cyst. The wrist is the prime site for ganglions, although they do occur elsewhere in the body. They are most frequently seen on the dorsum of the wrist, but occasionally occur on the palmar aspect, usually on the radial side. They are often seen in typists and keyboard operators where their cosmetic effect may be the chief complaint.

They vary in size and in the degree of pressure with which they are distended in parallel with the amount of activity of the wrist. A well established ganglion may disappear with rest and inactivity, only to recur months or years later. They tend to produce local pain and ache while they are developing, filling, and pushing their way up through the tissues, and the ganglion which is causing the most severe complaints may be the smallest and the most difficult to palpate.

The treatment of choice, if any treatment is warranted, is surgical excision after careful dissection of the entire cyst including its neck of origin from joint capsule or tendon sheath. Less painstaking excision, like the age-old treatment of simply breaking the cyst, preferrably with the family Bible, is likely to be followed by recurrence.

CARPAL TUNNEL SYNDROME (6)

The carpal tunnel on the palmar side of the wrist has already been described. Anything which increases the tissue mass within this rigid tunnel may produce compression neuritis of the median nerve. Among the causes may be swelling of the carpal joints, thickening of the flexor tendons or their sheaths, bony productive changes such as occur in degenerative arthritis or medical conditions producing generalized edema.

Pressure on the median nerve causes numbness and tingling in the thumb, index and middle fingers and, if unrelenting, atrophy of muscle in the ball of the thumb. Symptoms are aggravated by palmar-flexion of the wrist and tend to be worse at night, probably due to the fact that most people sleep with their wrists in this position. Symptoms become worse when the hand is in a dependent position as venous engorgement adds to the pressure within the carpal tunnel. The syndrome is fairly common in industry where it is often related to repetitive hand work. It is somewhat more common in women than in men.

Examination is frequently not very revealing unless the condition has been present long enough to produce the characteristic partial atrophy of muscle in the ball of the thumb. It is usually possible to duplicate or aggravate the complaints by holding the wrist in a position of full palmar flexion for 30 seconds or so. The definitive diagnostic test is an electromyogram and nerve conduction study which will show denervation potentials in the muscle and slowing of nerve conduction time.

Conservative treatment includes the use of night splints to prevent palmar flexion of the wrists during sleep and the use of anti-inflammatory medications. If generalized edema is present, medical treatment of the cause is indicated along with the use of diuretics. If the patient does repetitive hand work, a change of job may be helpful.

If conservative treatment fails, and the degree of disability warrants, surgical decompression of the carpal tunnel is done by transecting the carpal ligament. If symptoms have been of long duration, recovery is likely to be slow. The condition often occurs in the opposite wrist, indicating a fairly high degree of individual susceptibility. Permanent interdiction of repetitive hand work is probably wise in any patient with carpal tunnel syndrome.

CHAPTER 4
THE ELBOW (42)

Ostensibly a fairly simple hinge joint, the elbow is complicated by the structural design which allows for forearm rotation. The hinge function is served by the inner or medial half of the joint where the rounded medial condyle of the humerus is seated in a concavity in the upper end of the ulna (Figure 17). Rotation of the forearm takes place on the lateral side of the elbow where the round head of the radius articulates with the lateral humeral condyle, participating in the hinge motion, but capable of pivoting through an arc of 180 degrees.

Lateral support of the complex hinge is derived in part from two powerful muscle groups, one on the lateral side of the elbow, the other on the medial side. These muscles arise mainly from the small lateral and medial epicondyles of the humerus and cross the joint into the forearm, wrist and hand. The lateral group are extensors of the wrist and fingers and rotate the forearm into the palm-up position. The medial group flex the wrist and fingers and roll the forearm into the palm-down position.

The attachment of strong muscle groups into relatively limited bony areas may give rise to clinical problems because of the concentrated pull exerted by the muscle fibers ont the small area of the fibrous covering of the bone (periosteum) into which they insert. Mechanical irritation caused by heavy or prolonged use of such muscles occasionally evokes a secondary inflammatory reaction in this circumscribed point of attachment with resultant pain and disability (epicondylitis).

Forearm rotation deserves special mention since it is so vital to the efficient function of the hand and is threatened by wrist, elbow and forearm injuries. As the forearm lies in full supination with the palm facing upward, the forearm bones are parallel, the radius on the outer or lateral side at both elbow and wrist. As the forearm rolls into pronation with the palm facing downward, the radius crosses over the ulna and comes to lie on the inner or medial side of the forearm at the wrist, although it maintains its lateral position at the elbow. Maintaining full pronation and supination ranges is a primary consideration in the

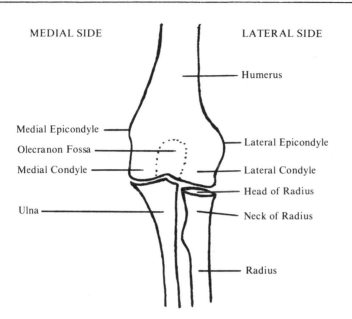

MEDIAL SIDE

LATERAL SIDE

Humerus

Medial Epicondyle

Olecranon Fossa

Medial Condyle

Ulna

Lateral Epicondyle

Lateral Condyle

Head of Radius

Neck of Radius

Radius

A. Antero-posterior view with elbow in full extension

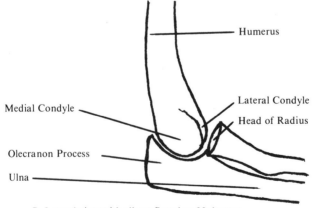

Humerus

Lateral Condyle

Head of Radius

Medial Condyle

Olecranon Process

Ulna

B. Lateral view with elbow flexed to 90 degrees

Figure 17. A. Antero-posterior view of left elbow in full extension.
B. Lateral view with elbow flexed to 90 degrees. The elbow joint includes
two articulations: the hinge joint between the proximal end of the ulna and
the medial condyle of the humerus, and the pivot joint between the head of
the radius and the lateral humeral condyle.

treatment of wrist, elbow and forearm injuries.

The fall on the outstretched hand poses a threat to the elbow. If the force of the upward thrust is not dissipated by fractures at the wrist level (carpal navicular or distal radius), it continues along the shaft of the radius and may exert its full impact at the elbow, driving the round, gently cupped head of the radius against the lateral condyle of the humerus and causing fractures of the head or neck of the radius.

The olecranon process forms the point of the elbow and is covered only by skin and subcutaneous tissue. It is subject to severe impact in the typical backward fall in which the body weight often lands on the back of the flexed elbow. Even resting the flexed elbow on a flat hard surface concentrates significant pressure upon the unpadded olecranon. Nature provides a degree of protection in the form of the olecranon bursa which lies between the sharp tip of the olecranon process and the skin. When subject to unusual friction or to bumping, the olecranon bursa may over-secrete lubricating fluid, become inflamed and thickened and require treatment.

When the elbow is fully extended, the olecranon process enters a bony hollow in the back of the humerus and the elbow is locked. Any further hyper-extension force may lever the humerus forward and out of articulation with the two forearm bones producing dislocation of the elbow. In the process, there may be fractures of the head or neck of the radius and of the front lip of the concavity in the upper ulna, the coronoid process. Extensive soft tissue damage threatening elbow stability always occurs. Elbow dislocations or subluxations are sometimes reduced at the site of injury, either spontaneously or with the help of by-standers, and their presence not made known to the first examiner on arrival at the treatment facility. It is important to obtain this information so that treatment may be modified to insure that joint stability is not lost.

Reasoning from the anatomy of the elbow, it is logical to predict a fairly high incidence of potentially serious fractures, an occasional dislocation, some special problems relating to the medial and lateral support musculature at the epicondyles and troubles in the region of the exposed olecranon process and its bursa.

FRACTURES (12)
Head of the radius (7)

If the upward impact from a fall on the outstretched hand passes the wrist without producing fracture there, it is transmitted along the shaft of the radius and drives the head of the radius into the lateral humeral condyle. The rounded condyle acts like a blunt chisel and may split the head of the radius longitudinally with varying degree of displacement of the bony fragments.

Undisplaced or minimally displaced radial head fractures (Figure 18) are treated with a light posterior plaster splint or, sometimes, with a simple elastic bandage wrap and a sling for a few days until the patient is comfortable and then mobilized as rapidly as possible. Exercises are directed at preserving and regaining full supination and extension, which are the motions most likely to be lost. The patient is encouraged, as soon as possible, to rest or read at intervals with the back of the elbow resting upon a small cushion so that the weight of the forearm will gradually stretch it into full extension. Forearm roll exercise can be carried out by having the patient hold a hammer by the end of its handle and allowing the weight of the hammer head to stretch the muscles into the full palm-up and palm-down positions. Active return of the hammer head to the neutral thumb-up position will provide alternate active exercise of the pronators and the supinators.

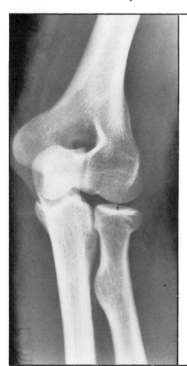

Figure 18. Typical "chisel" fracture of the head of the radius with no significant displacement.

The patient is encouraged to use the arm normally for day-to-day activities, but heavy work is interdicted for six to eight weeks. Although clinically healed and comfortable on full activity at about eight weeks, x-ray will often show an open fracture line for several months. This finding need not interfere with such activity as is comfortable.

If fractures of the head of the radius are severely displaced so that the articular surface is irregular, surgical resection of the radial head is carried out. Painless forearm roll is often better served by clearing the joint between the radial head and the lateral humeral condyle completely rather than leaving a rough and irregular radial head to grind away at the articulation. Ordinarily, about three-quarters of an inch of the radial head is removed and the collar-like ligament which binds the neck of the radius to the ulna is preserved.

The general rule of thumb for deciding which radial head fractures must be referred for consideration of surgery states that fractures resulting in depression of more than one-third of the articular surface by more than one-eighth of an inch will probably do better if the radial head is excised. Figure 19 shows a borderline case which might be

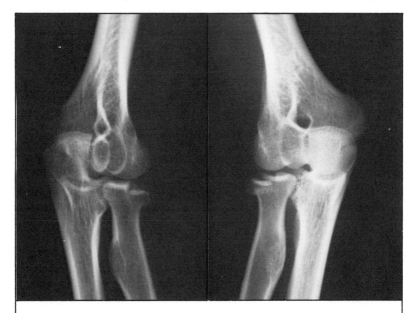

Figure 19. Displaced fracture of the head of the radius, borderline for closed or open treatment. About one-third of the radial head is displaced downward about one-eighth of an inch.

handled either way depending upon the age and functional requirements of the individual.

Neck of radius (2)

If the shock wave of transmitted force up the radial shaft is not directly head-on, a fracture through the narrow neck of the radius, more or less transverse in direction, may occur and the radial head may be angulated or, sometimes, popped off completely. Unless angulation is minimal and displacement virtually non-existant, as determined by comparable x-rays of the opposite elbow, expert opinion and treatment is indicated.

If fracture of the head or neck of the radius has been accompanied by dislocation of the elbow, as occasionally happens, the radius may have to be preserved as a stabilizer of the joint until soft tissue healing has occurred, regardless of the rule-of-thumb indications for excision. Sometimes, the dislocation is not reported when the patient arrives at the medical department and a fracture of the head or neck of the radius may be the only positive finding on initial evaluation, and it may be sufficiently displaced to warrant excision of the radial head. Lacking information as to the dislocation, surgical treatment may proceed and be followed by disastrous recurrent dislocation, chronic instability of the elbow, and a severe and permanent disability. Close inquiry of the patient and first aid people as to the immediate appearance of the elbow and any on-site manipulation to exclude the possibility of hidden dislocation or subluxation may be the salvation of an elbow.

Olecranon (2)

Most fractures of the olecranon break the process completely, enter the joint and are widely separated because of the pull of the triceps muscle which attaches to the proximal fragment. They will require open reduction and internal fixation.

Bony spurs frequently form near the tip of the olecranon process in the region of attachment of the triceps muscle and these may be fractured by a fall on the point of the elbow (1). They can be treated symptomatically and often unite by fibrous tissue rather than bone. Occasionally, local tenderness persists and the spur must be surgically excised for comfort.

Medial epicondyle of humerus (1)

Usually an avulsion fracture caused by the pull of the flexor-pronator group of muscles as the elbow subluxes or dislocates laterally, the small medial epicondyle is often incarcerated in the joint as the elbow spontaneously reduces. It may be difficult to recognize by x-ray. Comparable x-ray views of the normal elbow are helpful in the identification of this injury by revealing the altered bony contour of the medial side of the humerus where the epicondyle is missing on the injured side. The injury is more common in youth before complete closure of the epiphyseal line of the medial epicondyle but does occur in the industrial population and is important to recognize early. Surgery is necessary to extract the bony fragment and its attached muscles from within the joint.

EPICONDYLITIS (10)
Lateral epicondylitis (10)

Also known as tennis elbow, pitcher's elbow or bowler's elbow, lateral epicondylitis represents a combination of mechanical irritation from the pull of the extensor-supinator muscles upon the small area of periosteum of the lateral epicondyle plus a secondary inflammatory reaction. Symptoms may follow a single direct blow, but more commonly result from repeated strain.

On examination, patients show severe local tenderness over the lateral epicondyle with pain in this area when the extensor-supinator muscles of the forearm are passively stretched by flexing the wrist and fingers and bringing the forearm into the full palm-down position with the elbow extended. Alternatively, there is pain the same region when the patient actively extends the wrist and fingers and rolls the forearm into palm-up position against resistance.

Successful treatment is usually a combination of anti-inflammatory and mechanical approaches. Anti-inflammatory measures may include the use of systemic medications such as phenyl butazone or local injection of steroids directly into the area of maximum tenderness. Mechanical treatment seeks to relieve the pull of the extensor-supinator muscles upon the inflamed periosteum. It may include limitation or modification of activity, the use of a cock-up splint for the wrist, wearing of a snug non-elastic band about the forearm and, as symptoms abate, corrective exercises. The symptomatic tennis player may need some coaching in backhand swing and an alteration in the grip of the racket, along with anti-inflammatory medication.

The application of local heat or ultrasound has not been strikingly effective in most cases and occasionally will aggravate the symptoms. In the rare and extreme case, surgical release of the extensor-supinator muscles from the lateral epicondyle may have to be done.

Medial epicondylitis (*)

Identical in nature to lateral epicondylitis except that the attachment of the flexor-pronator muscles into the medial epicondyle is involved, medial epicondylitis is less common. Clinical findings are reversed, passive stretch of the flexors and pronators causing pain, as does active flexion of the wrist and fingers and pronation of the forearm against resistance. Treatment is similar to that for lateral epicondylitis except that local injection is undertaken with more caution because of the position of the ulnar nerve immediately behind the medial epicondyle.

OLECRANON BURSITIS (20)

Following a single impact, the olecranon bursa is usually distended with blood and is treated by aspiration and the application of a compression bandage. With repeated irritation, the contents of the bursa will more likely be a clear serous fluid and, even after aspiration, there may be palpable thickening of the bursal walls. Usually, local steroids are injected into the bursa after aspiration and a compression dressing is applied in an effort to prevent recurrent effusion. Recurrences are common, however, and repeated aspiration and injection may be necessary. If the condition is not controlled after three or so such treatments, surgical excision of the chronically inflamed bursal sac may be necessary.

Chronic olecranon bursitis is fairly often associated with an olecranon spur and, if this is present, it should be excised along with the bursa. Chronic bursitis not clearly related to mechanical irritation should be studied to exclude gout or one of the arthritides.

CHAPTER 5
THE SHOULDER (53)

Nowhere in the body is the option for mobility over stability more clearly articulated than in the shoulder joint. Capable of a range of 180 degrees in bringing the arm away from the side and into the overhead position (abduction), the shoulder can also produce about 180 degrees of rotation of the arm relative to the long axis of the body and a grand arc of 240 degrees in forward and backward elevation.

So great is the degree of mobility that the shoulder is stabilized almost exclusively by tendons rather than by the mechanical fit of the opposing bones or by snug ligaments. More saucer than socket, the glenoid process of the scapula has a surface only about one-eighth as large as the globular head of the humerus (Figure 20). Apart from some thickened bands in the baggy capsule of the joint which check the extremes of motion, there are no ligaments worthy of the name.

Several tendons perform double duty as both movers and stabilizers of the joint and, since they constitute the meat of the story of the clinical problems of the shoulder, they should be placed in mind with relation to the bony landmarks of the shoulder area sketched in Figure 20.

Perhaps the most important is a conjoined sheet of three tendons, collectively known as the rotator cuff, which attach into the ridge of the greater tuberosity like a hood across the top 180 degrees of the shoulder. From front to back, these are the supraspinatus, the infraspinatus and the teres minor. The muscle bellies of all lie along the back surface of the scapula. The flat tendons of these three muscles pass beneath the overhanging arch made by the acromion process and the clavicle and fuse into a continuous sheet of tendon tissue before anchoring into the greater tuberosity. As movers, they rotate the humeral head on the glenoid and initiate the motion of abduction. Once motion of the arm away from the side has been started by the rotator cuff tendons, the full range of abduction is accomplished by the deltoid muscle which caps and gives contour to the shoulder area. The rotator cuff then simply provides a kind of fulcrum action, holding the head of the humerus against the glenoid to provide mechanical advantage for the deltoid.

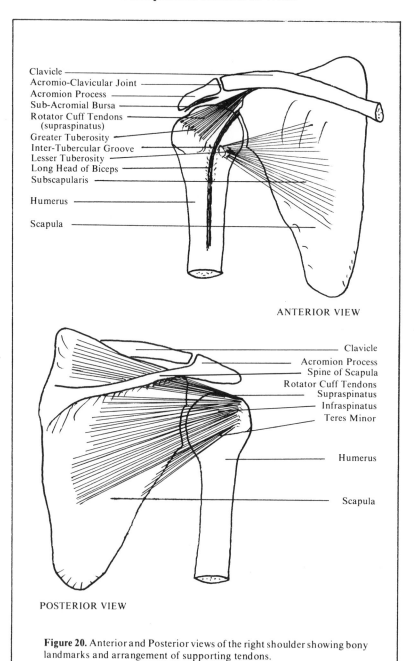

Clavicle
Acromio-Clavicular Joint
Acromion Process
Sub-Acromial Bursa
Rotator Cuff Tendons
   (supraspinatus)
Greater Tuberosity
Inter-Tubercular Groove
Lesser Tuberosity
Long Head of Biceps
Subscapularis

Humerus

Scapula

ANTERIOR VIEW

Clavicle
Acromion Process
Spine of Scapula
Rotator Cuff Tendons
Supraspinatus
Infraspinatus
Teres Minor

Humerus

Scapula

POSTERIOR VIEW

Figure 20. Anterior and Posterior views of the right shoulder showing bony landmarks and arrangement of supporting tendons.

Without the rotator cuff, the head of the humerus would drop out of the glenoid saucer.

As the arm is brought away from the side and into the overhead position, the rotator cuff tendons and the bony ridge of the greater tuberosity must pass beneath the bony arch made up by the acromion and the clavicle. Clearance is tight, friction of tendon or bone against the underside of the arch is possible, and nature has interposed a bursa, known as the sub-acromial or sub-deltoid bursa as a friction preventer. Like all bursae, it occupies but microscopic space under normal conditions. Irritation of this bursa with over-secretion of fluid or inflammation with thickening of the bursal walls, however, may exceed the scant space tolerance and make it painful or impossible to bring the arm away from the side more than a few degrees.

Stabilization of a different nature is supplied by the tendon of the long head of the biceps. From its muscle belly on the front of the upper arm, this tendon passes upward, enters the valley between the greater tuberosity ridge and the lesser tuberosity, arches over the head of the humerus and attaches into the top lip of the glenoid. The valley between the tuberosities (intertubercular groove) is converted into a tunnel by a roofing ligament and the humerus is quite literally strung upon the tendon of the long head of the biceps like a bead on a string.

Tendon tissue is apparently physiologically ill-suited for the stabilizing duties ordinarily assigned to ligaments and the shoulder tendons which perform as stabilizers of the joint begin to show attritional changes around age 25. Degenerative changes in the support tendons of the shoulder and the reaction of surrounding tissues to those changes form the pathomechanical basis for many of the common clinical conditions about the shoulder.

One other stabilizing tendon should be placed. The subscapularis muscle lies along the front or inner surface of the scapula. Its tendon winds around the front of the shoulder joint and attaches into the lesser tuberosity. It is the main buttress of the shoulder joint against the common anterior dislocation and, in most operations for recurrent dislocation, the subscapularis tendon is reefed or double-breasted to increase its stabilizing effect.

In addition to the shoulder joint itself (gleno-humeral joint), the acromio-clavicular joint lies in the shoulder region and is subject to injury, usually by falls on the tip of the shoulder.

FRACTURES (5)

Because of its high mobility and the semi-elastic nature of its tendon support mechanisms, fractures about the shoulder are not common in the age groups making up the industrial population. Neither fracture of the clavicle, which is quite common in youth, nor fracture of the neck of the humerus, a fairly frequent injury of the elderly, is statistically represented in the sampling of industrial orthopaedic injuries.

Avulsion fracture of the greater tuberosity (4) occurs as the patient, starting to fall to the side, makes a sudden violent move to abduct his arm and cushion the impact. The rotator cuff tendons, initiators of abduction, may tear or they may rip off a portion of the greater tuberosity ridge into which they insert. The avulsed fragment usually involves only a portion of the greater tuberosity and is not widely displaced. The injury can be treated symptomatically much like a partial tear of the rotator cuff. Sling fixation is used for the minimum time necessary to obtain relief of pain and shoulder motion is then started and advanced as rapidly as tolerated.

Early shoulder motion in this and other painful conditions of the shoulder can comfortably be undertaken with pendulum exercises. The patient, leaning forward 90 degrees from a standing position, rests his well arm on a table or chair back for support and allows the injured arm to dangle vertically. In this position, the arm can be swung forward and backward, away from the body and across the body, and rotated with little discomfort. Holding a flat-iron or similar object in the hand makes the pendulum exercises even more comfortable and provides some resistance against which to exercise the muscles.

Fracture of the body of the scapula (1) occurs from a direct blow on the back, often from a falling object. The fracture is usually comminuted but, since the scapula lies completely within a muscle envelope, not significantly displaced. Healing is generally prompt.

DISLOCATIONS (9)

Most dislocations are anterior, the head of the humerus being forced out the front of the joint and then dropping downward (Figure 21). They usually result from force applied to the abducted arm, either in a fall or by some major impact. The quarterback, his arm cocked to pass, is a shoulder dislocation waiting to happen as he is stormed by defensive linemen and the occasional blitzing linebacker.

If seen soon after injury, most dislocations can be reduced fairly readily by placing the patient face down on a table with the injured arm

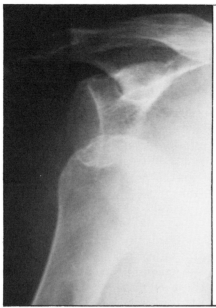

Figure 21. Typical anterior dislocation of the shoulder. The head of the humerus lies below and in front of the glenoid.

dangling over the side. If muscle relaxation can be obtained, either by pain medication or by the confidence of the patient in the attendant, gentle downward traction on the arm will often produce reduction. Occasionally, the upper humerus must be levered gently outward and toward the patient's head.

If x-rays have not been made before reduction, in the interests of the earliest and easiest reduction maneuver, they should be made after reduction to confirm positioning and to exclude other injury.

If immediate reduction cannot be achieved, the patient should be referred for expert hospital treatment. Reduction may be blocked by associated fractures in the area or simply by the amount of elapsed time since injury and the resultant muscle spasm in the area. General anaesthesia is likely to be necessary to effect reduction.

A complete x-ray examination of the shoulder including antero-posterior, lateral and axillary views will be necessary to assess the situation. In addition to revealing possible fractures, these views are necessary to detect the occasional posterior dislocation which may be missed in a routine antero-posterior view.

After reduction, the shoulder is immobilized in a sling with a body swathe wrapped over the sling and around the chest wall for periods varying from three to six weeks depending upon estimation of the risk of recurrent dislocation.

Recurrent dislocation (4) represents a real threat in any shoulder dislocation, but is especially frequent in younger patients. Recent studies indicate that, if the first dislocation occurs before age 20, recurrent dislocation is likely in 90 percent of patients. Between ages 20 and 40, the recurrence rate is about 70 percent. After age 40, the risk of recurrent dislocation drops to around 15 percent.

The higher the statistical risk of recurrent dislocation, the longer should be the period of post reduction immobilization. Fortunately, younger patients with the highest risk tolerate long periods of immobilization and regain shoulder motion easily. Older patients who tolerate immobilization less well are at lower risk and may be mobilized earlier.

Recurrent dislocations reduce more easily than do first dislocations, progressively so with the number of dislocations. They also occur more easily to the point that the patient with established recurrent dislocation may pop the shoulder out by turning over in bed. When frequency of recurrent dislocation becomes a disability, the patient should be referred for surgical repair. A number of procedures are available and are generally quite successful in stabilizing the shoulder. They may produce some permanent loss of the terminal ranges of abduction and external rotation.

TENDINITIS (26)
Rotator cuff tendinitis (23)
Also known as supraspinatus tendinitis, subdeltoid bursitis, subacromial bursitis or partial tear of the rotator cuff, the basic pathology begins with degenerative changes in the rotator cuff tendons, most predominantly in the supraspinatus and usually more marked in the dominant side shoulder.

Because of the relative avascularity of tendons, attritional changes cannot be repaired and become cumulative. The unusual stabilizing function thrust upon the rotator cuff tendons renders them unduly susceptible to such changes, and they begin early in life. Everyday use of the shoulder, along with the usual assortment of minor injuries, produce microscopic tears and ravelings of tendon fibers near their insertion into the greater tuberosity and gradually result in thickening and nubbiness of the tendon.

The subacromial bursa is rubbed and abraded between the rough and thickened tendon and the bony undersurface of the acromion as the arm is used in abduction and rotation and responds, as do all irritated bursae, by over-secretion of lubricating fluid and thickening of its walls. Increased tissue mass in this confined space causes more friction, friction causes irritation and still more thickening of the bursa, and the vicious cycle sets the stage for the onset of symptoms.

Symptoms, often very severe, may be precipitated by a single injury, by repetitive motions of the arm involving abduction or rotation, or may appear spontaneously. Whatever the mode of onset, symptoms usually result from an inflammatory process. Granulation tissue, the stuff of healing, which carries a copious blood and nerve supply, invades the area of attritional changes and, if sufficient in degree and duration, may repair the accumulation of micro damage in the tendon.

The hotter the inflammatory reaction, the greater the pain. On the other hand, the more acute the shoulder symptoms, the better the prognosis. Acute shoulders with extremely severe pain nearly always recover, almost regardless of treatment, in about three weeks. Chronic, low-grade shoulder symptoms are likely to be slow to subside.

The typical patient with rotator cuff tendinitis has pain in the front of the shoulder accentuated by any attempt to abduct the arm away from the side more than a few degrees. Rotation of the arm, especially internal rotation, as in reaching behind into a hip pocket or hooking a bra, is likely to be painful or impossible. Reaching upwards in front (forward elevation) is uncomfortable, but not as painful nor as restricted as abduction and internal rotation.

In supraspinatus tendinitis, the most common form, there is tenderness to palpation, more or less localized, over the front of the shoulder an inch or so lateral to the front border of the deltoid muscle and just beneath the outer end of the clavicle. Patients with severe inflammatory reactions involving the subacromial bursa as well as the tendon may show diffuse tenderness over the entire anterior and lateral aspects of the shoulder and there may be increased local heat in the area.

In less acute situations, the patient may be able to abduct the arm to 90 degrees, but can seldom accomplish full abduction range, and usually has pain with rotation when the arm is abducted to the horizontal position. Crepitus can often be felt and heard as rotation in the position of 90 degrees of abduction rubs the inflamed tendon and bursa between the greater tuberosity and the overhanging ledge of the acromion.

Treatment consists of control of the inflammatory reaction and preservation of shoulder motion. If tenderness is well localized, injection of steroids into the area of maximum tenderness can produce dramatic relief. If symptoms are severe, indicative of a massive inflammatory reaction, but tenderness is diffuse, a short course of systemic steroids or of non-steroid anti-inflammatory drugs may be effective.

Chronic tendinitis with low-grade symptoms usually requires long term mangement. Salicylate compounds in regular dosage may be the drugs of choice to control the smouldering inflammatory reaction. An exercise program, beginning with pendulum exercises, and advancing to abduction exercises must be instituted and patiently supervised. Physiotherapy, if available, is useful in these patients and a dedicated physiotherapist can do much to shorten the course and minimize the disability.

Calcification may occur in the degenerating tendons and be visable by x-ray. While confirmatory of the diagnosis of tendinitis, its presence is largely incidental and does not imply any alteration of the basic pathological process or indication for modification of treatment. Some judgement may be made as to the duration and progression of the condition by the appearance of the calcified deposit in the x-ray. Smooth-edged, rounded, high-density deposits have generally been present for months or years, often long before the onset of symptoms. Soft, cottony, low-density calcification is more likely to be recent in origin and may be absorbed during the period of symptoms and treatment. Sometimes the deposit is seen distal to the tendons' insertion into the greater tuberosity, indicating that the deposit has ruptured through from the tendon, where it originated, into the subacromial bursa.

If, after a significant injury, there is complete inability to initiate abduction of the shoulder, a major rupture of the rotator cuff tendons should be suspected and the patient referred for opinion as to whether surgical repair of the tendon is indicated. Apart from major ruptures of the rotator cuff, the surgical treatment of tendinitis has not been outstandingly successful.

Bicipital tenditis (3)

Tendinitis similar to that of the rotator cuff tendons may occur in the long head of the biceps, usually in the area of its passage through the intertubercular tunnel. In bicipital tendinitis, the point of maximum tenderness lies over the groove between the greater and lesser tuberosities, a little medial to the usual point of tenderness found in supraspinatus tendinitis. The patient has pain on forward elevation of the arm as well as on abduction. The crucial diagnostic sign of bicipital tendinitis is pain on supination of the forearm against resistance, even when the shoulder is immobile at the side. This pain is accurately referred to the bicipital groove along the front of the shoulder and is due to the fact that biceps muscle is a powerful supinator of the forearm. Treatment follows the lines suggested for rotator cuff tendinitis.

Any type of tendinitis in the shoulder area may, in certain patients, give rise to the "frozen shoulder" syndrome characterized by extremely severe and intractable pain of a causalgic nature, evidence of neuro-vascular dysfunction involving the entire upper extremity, and total loss of all shoulder motion. Even the suspicion of true frozen shoulder is reason for immediate referral of the patient for the most expert care available. Treatment is difficult, may involve sympathetic nerve blocks and other sophisticated modalities, and the earlier instituted the better.

RUPTURE OF THE LONG HEAD OF THE BICEPS (5)

Subject, like the rotator cuff tendons, to early attritional changes and tendinitis, the long head of the biceps suffers the added mechanical disadvantage of enclosure in a rigid bony tunnel for several inches of its length. Degenerative changes may become so severe that the tendon ruptures. Such ruptures usually occur in the 40 to 60 year age group, sometimes with normal use, but often when there is sudden and unexpected loading of the biceps, as in attempting to catch a falling object. Patients experience momentary pain at the instant of rupture but, if the rupture is complete, are not thereafter particularly uncomfortable. They may often be more concerned with the "Pop-Eye" bulge of the biceps contour of the upper arm. Partial tears occasionally occur and often are more painful than complete ruptures.

Surgical repair may be indicated depending upon the age and functional demands of the patient, and upon the severity of the psychological reaction to the abnormal appearance of the arm. Normal or nearly normal function is usually regained whether the rupture is repaired or not.

SPRAINS (4)

Sprains generally involve the acromio-clavicular ligaments and result from falls on the tip of the shoulder. Mild sprains (2) do not affect the integrity of the acromio-clavicular joint and can be treated symptomatically with a sling for a few days until the shoulder is comfortable. They do not threaten permanency. Severe sprains (2) of the acromio-clavicular ligaments produce variable degrees of instability of the acromio-clavicular joint, known as shoulder separation. The joint may be widened or, with more severe injury, there may be upward displacement of the outer end of the clavicle.

Widening of the acromio-clavicular joint may be detected as a palpable gap between the end of the clavicle and the acromion if the patient is seen soon after injury. Significant upward displacement of the outer end of the clavicle is easily visable and palpable. As in all sprains, it becomes the responsibility of the examiner to determine the degree of instability of the joint.

Routine x-rays of the shoulder, made in the recumbent position, may fail to reveal abnormality of the acromio-clavicular joint after sprain and it is necessary to make stress films to determine the degree of instability, if any. These x-rays are made with the patient sitting upright, holding a weight in each hand, with the shoulder muscles relaxed. Antero-posterior views of both shoulders are made and the injured

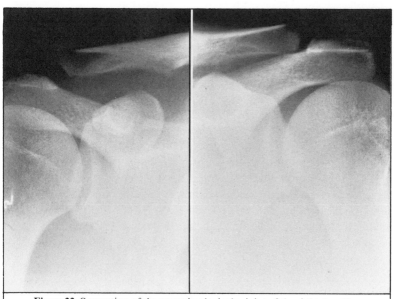

Figure 22. Separation of the acromio-clavicular joint of the right shoulder (viewer's left) with slight upward displacement of clavicle. X-rays were made in the upright position with downward traction on both arms. Routine shoulder x-rays made in the recumbent position showed no abnormality.

shoulder is compared with the normal. In moderate sprains, the joint on the injured side will be widened (Figure 22). In severe sprains, there will be upward displacement of the clavicle.

Unless the acromio-clavicular joint is totally disrupted with the outer end of the clavicle displaced well above the acromion, in which case surgical repair may be indicated, most acromio-clavicular separations are treated in a high sling, well padded where it crosses the back of the neck, which supports the entire weight of the arm. Beyond this, no serious attempt is made to reduce the displacement. The joint is protected in this fashion for three to four weeks and the shoulder is then mobilized. Most patients do quite well, even though there may be residual displacement of the outer end of the clavicle.

Occasionally, traumatic arthritis of the acromio-clavicular joint may develop and, for some patients who regularly perform overhead work, may present enough of a problem to warrant surgical intervention. This generally involves resection of the distal inch or so of the clavicle to clear the joint of further friction irritation from the displaced clavicle.

STRAINS (3)

Most shoulder strains are minor tears of the rotator cuff tendons which do not evoke the inflammatory reaction which would lead to a diagnosis of tendinitis. They are generally treated symptomatically with attention to the preservation of the mobility of the shoulder and present no great problem.

CHAPTER 6
THE FOOT (139)

An assembly of 26 bones snugly bound together by strong ligaments, the foot has limited flexibility, at least in non-tropical shoe-wearing societies. It does have the capacity to tilt from side to side and thus adapt to uneven or sloping surfaces, and the presence of longitudinal and transverse arches provides some shock absorbing effect. In terms of active motion, it contributes some power to the push-off phase of the gait.

The longitudinal arch along the inner side of the foot (Figure 23) contributes some springiness. This dorsally bowed convexity arcs from the ball of the foot to the bottom of the heel and is maintained by a bow-string ligament bridging between the metatarsal heads and the calcaneus. There is also a kind of arch across the forepart of the foot where weight bearing is mainly concentrated beneath the heads of the first and fifth metatarsals and the second, third and fourth metatarsal heads bear only token weight. Collapse of this transverse or metatarsal arch gives rise to at least as many clinical problems as does flattening of the longitudinal arch.

Adaptability of the foot to the slope of the surface upon which it is placed depends upon the ability of the foot to tilt inwards and outwards and this is a function of the joint between the calcaneus and the talus (Figure 23). This joint is called the sub-talar or sub-astragalar joint and pain or loss of motion in this joint can be extremely disabling for the standing or walking worker especially if the work is on uneven ground or sloping surfaces. The nomenclature for this important tilting motion of the foot is confusing. Inclination of the sole of the foot inward toward the midline of the body is variously called inversion, adduction or supination. Angling the sole of the foot outward away from the midline is termed eversion, abduction or pronation. Inversion and eversion seem to be the simplest and most meaningful terms and will be used in this text.

In forced inversion or eversion motion which exceeds the limited range of the sub-talar joint (about 25 degrees of inversion and about 15

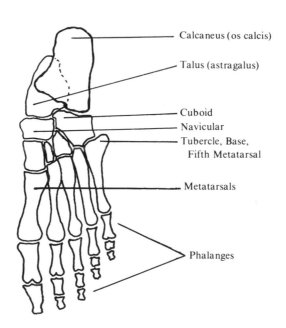

Calcaneus (os calcis)

Talus (astragalus)

Cuboid
Navicular
Tubercle, Base,
  Fifth Metatarsal

Metatarsals

Phalanges

A. Bones of the tarsus and foot viewed from below

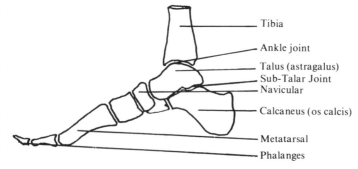

Tibia

Ankle joint

Talus (astragalus)
Sub-Talar Joint
Navicular

Calcaneus (os calcis)

Metatarsal
Phalanges

B. Side view of ankle, tarsus and foot

Figure 23. Bones of the tarsus and foot. Scheme of nomenclature of foot bones is similar to that of hand bones. The seven tarsal bones are intrinsic to foot structure and function and are considered a part of the foot.

degrees of eversion), the force is transmitted through to the ankle joint and is a potent cause of injury at that level.

Rotation of the foot relative to the lower leg is similarly limited. A few degrees are allowed at the ankle joint and a little rotation can be produced in the tarsal joints, mainly those between the calcaneus and cuboid and between the talus and navicular (Figure 23). Tarsal rotation, however, is pretty much eliminated by a firm-soled shoe and excessive forced motion in the rotation range will usually be passed through to the ankle joint with the potentiality for injury there. Most ankle injuries result from a combination of inversion and internal rotation or of eversion and external rotation which exceed the limited capabilities of the foot to absorb them.

As might be anticipated, the foot is extremely vulnerable to fractures, both by direct violence and from forced motion which exceeds the limited range of its tightly supported joints. Because of the close relationship of the bones, multiple fractures often result from a single injury and the Frequency Index for fractures of the foot (141) actually exceeds the Frequency Index for the entire foot (139).

FRACTURES (141)

Nearly 80 percent of all foot fractures involve the toes and almost all of them could be prevented by the wearing of safety shoes since they lie within the area protected by the metal toe cap.

Distal Phalanx (88)

Distal phalanx fractures of the toes, like those of the fingers, usually result from a crush injury, often from a falling object. They are somewhat less likely to be compound that those in the fingers. Toes have the same closed distal phalangeal compartment as do fingers and the pressure of traumatic exudate within this compartment may produce severe pain and require venting by puncturing the nail. No special fracture care is necessary and healing is usually prompt. Protection of the injured toe from irritation while healing may require a cut-out shoe or an orthopaedic clog. The risk of infection in compound fractures is a little higher in toes than in fingers because of foot moisture and tissue maceration and, in the older patient, because of diminished blood supply. Generally, they should be observed more carefully and dressings changed frequently in an effort to keep the area dry.

The distribution of distal phalanx fractures in toes shows a heavy predilection for great toe injury.

Great toe	60	Fourth toe	5
Second toe	7	Fifth toe	10
Third toe	6		

Middle Phalanx (2) and Proximal Phalanx (21)
The phalanges are shorter in the foot and the intrinsic musculature not as strong nor as well developed as in the hand. Consequently, there is less likelihood of angulation or displacement of middle and proximal phalanx fractures of toes. Except for the proximal phalanx of the great toe, most fractures can be treated by strapping the injured toe to the adjoining well toe, interposing a gauze pad between the toes to prevent maceration. Healing time is about three weeks. A normal shoe can usually be worn and the sole of the shoe gives added support and protection.
Because of the important thrust imparted by the great toe to the take-off phase of the gait, fractures of the proximal phalanx of the big toe require more rigid splinting and protection for a longer period of time. It may be necessary to use a wooden-soled orthopaedic clog to insure rigidity and immobilization during the healing period.
Infrequently, in the smaller toes, malunion with plantar angulation may create a bony prominence on the under surface of the toe which causes pain on weight bearing. If symptoms warrant, the phalanx may be excised without significant residual disability.

Metatarsal (22)

Fractures of the shafts of metatarsals (14) usually result from crush injuries and the degree of soft tissue damage may be as important a consideration in treatment as the fracture. Hemorrhage beneath the strong dorsal aponeurosis of the foot may so increase the pressure in the deeper parts of the foot as to threaten the arterial supply to the toes. The familiar triad of ice, compression and elevation is used, but under close observation with frequent checks of circulation in the toes. Special caution is warranted in older patients who may have some degree of occlusive arterial disease.
Fractures of the shaft of the great toe metatarsal (7) usually require rigid fixation in a plaster boot because of the importance of the first metatarsal as a pillar of the longitudinal arch and because of the heavy share of body weight which it bears. Cast application is best deferred until soft tissue swelling has been brought under control. No weight

bearing is allowed for the first three to four weeks. Another three to four weeks is then spent in a walking cast.

Fractures of the second, third and fourth metatarsal shafts (7) are usually stable because of intact neighboring metatarsals and the firm soft tissues interlacing the bones. Once soft tissue swelling has been controlled, these patients can often be allowed to walk with only the support of an elastic bandage and a shoe. Healing time is four to eight weeks.

Fractures of the base of the fifth metatarsal (7) are avulsion fractures. The prominent tubercle on the outer side of the base of the fifth metatarsal is the site of attachment of two peroneal muscles, which produce eversion of the foot. When the foot is twisted into inversion in the same kind of injury which often results in ankle sprain, the bony attachment of the peroneal muscles may be pulled off (Figure 24). There seldom is much displacement, although the avulsed fragment may be sizeable. Treatment is determined by the severity of symptoms. Some patients will require immobilization in a plaster boot for comfort. Most, however do well with a simple adhesive or elastic support once the

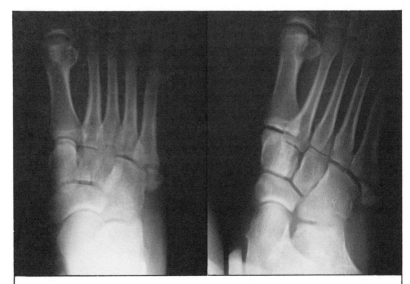

Figure 24. Antero-posterior and oblique views of the foot showing fracture of the base of the fifth metatarsal. This is an avulsion fracture of the insertions of the peroneal muscles produced by forcible inversion of the foot.

swelling has subsided. They may be allowed weight bearing in a shoe as soon as this is tolerable. Most have resumed full activity with comfort in three weeks or so, generally some time before bony healing of the fracture is demonstrated by x-ray.

March fracture (1) usually occurs in the slender neck of the second or third metatarsal and is a fatigue or insufficiency fracture. Patients complain of severe pain and tenderness over the mid-part of the forefoot, just back of the metatarsal heads, and generally have no history of accident. Frequently, there is a story of some unusual amount of activity on the feet - a long hike, an extended shopping trip in high heels, or early season jogging on hard surfaces.

   X-rays made within a few days of the onset of pain will usually be negative (Figure 25A) and the patient may be dismissed with a diagnosis of metatarsalgia. X-ray re-examination after three or four weeks, however, will show a fracture line across the narrow neck of the metatarsal and an impressive amount of callus (Figure 25B). So striking may be the appearance of the fresh, cottony healing bone tissue that diagnoses of bone tumor have been made by those unfamiliar with the

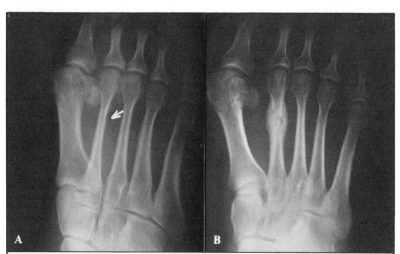

Figure 25. Insufficiency or "march fracture" of the neck of the second metatarsal. View on the left (A) is an antero-posterior view of the foot made two days after the onset of pain. Arrow indicates the slender neck of the metatarsal where unseen fracture has occurred. X-ray on the right (B) was made three weeks later and shows massive callus about the site of the fracture.

typical behavior of march fracture.

Treatment is symptomatic, but symptoms may persist for several months. They are better tolerated if a definite diagnosis has been made and the patient can be assured that the pain will finally disappear.

Calcaneus (5)

The heel bone (calcaneus, os calcis) is the site of two quite different types of fractures. Avulsion fractures result when one of the many ligaments attaching to the calaneus, with severe stretch, pulls off its insertion into the bone rather than tearing. Except for the anatomical details of the tissue injury, they are really sprains, and are treated as such. The second and much more important type of fracture is the crushing of the bone which is usually caused by a fall from a height, the patient landing on one or both feet.

Crush fractures (3) are important injuries because they often produce irregularity of the calcaneal surface of the sub-talar joint and, unless well managed, may result in a rigid, painful foot and a high degree of functional impairment. There is seldom much difficulty with the diagnosis and disposition of the severely comminuted and displaced calcaneus fractures. They are obvious by x-ray and should be immediately referred for expert treatment. Generally, an attempt is made to restore the contour of the bone and the all-important sub-talar articular surface by closed manipulation, with or without skeletal pin traction. This is often impossible and surgical arthrodesis of the sub-talar joint must be carried out to avoid a disablingly painful foot.

Much more troublesome both from the standpoint of diagnosis and of disposition are the milder crush fractures of the calcaneus. Fracture lines may be hard to see in the x-ray and the alteration in the contour of the bone is easy to miss. Since the injuries are often bilateral, there may be no opposite normal bone with which to compare. It is useful in such cases to check the tuber angle (Bohler's angle) on the lateral view x-ray of the heel (Figure 26). The dorsal surface of the calcaneus is normally tented upward toward the talus. This dorsal pointing angle can be best visualized by drawing two lines on the x-ray film. The first connects the highest middle prominence with the peak of the tuberosity on the posterior aspect of the calcaneus. The second connects the middle prominence with the most anterior bony prominence at the calcaneo-cuboid joint. The two lines should intersect at an angle of 30 degrees. Significant crush of the calcaneus will flatten, or even reverse, the tuber

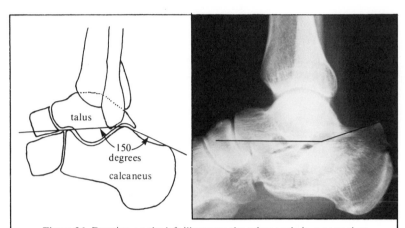

Figure 26. Drawing on the left illustrates the tuber angle in a normal os calcis. Lateral view x-ray of the heel on the right shows no clear-cut fracture lines, but the tuber angle has been reversed, signifying fracture of the os calcis with severe damage to the sub-talar joint.

angle and translates to significant alteration of the contour of the joint surface between the calcaneus and the talus.

Further assistance in identifying the more subtle calcaneal crush fractures is offered by a special x-ray view which allows the heel bone to be visualized in its cross-sectional contour. This view, known as the ski-jumper view, will detect bursting and lateral widening of the calcaneus. It is made by having the patient stand on the x-ray film with knees and hips flexed as if about to jump (Figure 27). The x-ray tube is just behind the patient and is aimed at an angle of 150 degrees from the vertical toward the forepart of the foot. If the patient is unable to stand, a similar, but somewhat less satisfactory view, can be obtained by placing the feet, heels down, on the x-ray film and having the patient pull the feet into maximum dorsi-flexion with a loop of gauze wrapped around both fore-feet. The x-ray tube is angled 30 degrees from the vertical toward the patient's head. Figure 28 shows a subtle calcaneus crush not easily identified in the routine lateral view, but producing definite alteration in the contour of the bone as seen in the ski-jumper view.

Calcaneal fractures with any degree of alteration of contour of the bone deserve expert care and carry a guarded prognosis with regard to the future painless function of the foot.

Avulsion fractures (2) most commonly involve the antero-superior

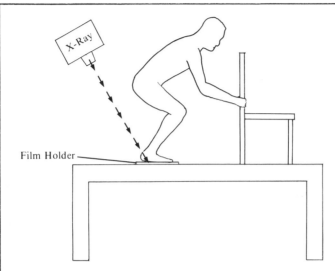

Figure 27. Position for axial view of calcaneal bones (ski-jumper view). Patient stands on the film holder on the x-ray table. Keeping the feet flat on the film holder, patient bends forward as if to jump, using a chair for support. Tube is angled 30 degrees off the vertical, centered on the heels.

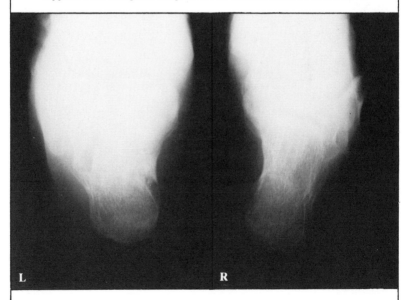

Figure 28. Axial ("ski-jumper") views of both heels. Broadening of the left os calcis is seen, indicative of crush fracture.

corner of the outer side of the heel bone in the region of attachment of the calcaneo-cuboid or talo-calcaneal ligaments. They follow inversion injury and can be treated as sprains with no great threat of permanency.

Other Tarsal Bone Fractures (3)

Avulsion fractures of the dorsal cortex of the head or neck of the talus or of the tarsal navicular occur in plantar flexion injuries of the foot. A common history is that, in descending a flight of stairs, the heel catches on the edge of a stair tread, the foot is forced downward into plantar flexion, and the patient may end up sitting on the heel. The dorsal ligaments connecting the talus and the navicular are torn loose at one or another of their insertions (Figure 29).

Treatment follows the routine for sprains. The avulsed fragments are ordinarily small but may be fairly widely separated from their bony beds, and often proceed to fibrous rather than bony union. There is rarely any significant degree of permanency.

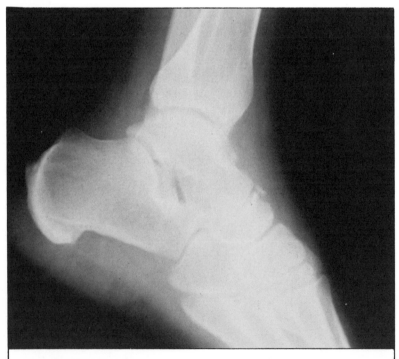

Figure 29. Lateral view of foot showing avulsion of a chip of bone from the dorsum of the tarsal navicular.

Talus (*)

Fractures of the talus, often accompanied by dislocations of the head of the talus and the navicular, or even of the whole talus, result from extreme inversion violence to the foot. The foot is usually medially displaced on the leg, severly inverted, and abnormal bony prominences can be seen and felt along its lateral side. There may be severe tenting of the skin over the lateral instep, or the skin may actually have burst, sometimes with extrusion of part or all of the talus. These injuries are obviously serious and are referred to the hospital and specialist care as emergencies.

SPRAINS (3)

Foot sprains are relatively uncommon. They usually result from inversion injuries and involve one or more of the tarsal joints. Chronic instability is seldom a threat and they generally can be treated symptomatically.

CONTUSIONS (3)

Occasionally, a crush of the foot by a heavy but large and rounded object such as an automobile tire may not cause fractures, but may, nevertheless, produce sufficient soft tissue bruising to lead to significant hemorrhage and tissue ooze deep within the foot. The firm dorsal aponeurosis may contain the mounting pressure until the arterial supply to the toes is threatened. The fact that the injured foot does not look particularly swollen, at least on the top, and that the x-rays are negative for fracture may lull the examiner into the belief that only minor injury has been sustained.

Along with routine measures to control the swelling, the circulation to the toes must be watched closely for at least the first 48 hours. Severe pain, discoloration and loss of capillary refill after compression of the toes may force emergency incision of the dorsal aponeurosis to relieve the pressure and prevent gangrene of the toes. Potentially dangerous at any age, the foot crush is especially so in patients over the age of 50.

Contusions of the ball of the foot or of the bottom of the heel may lead to long periods of painful weight bearing (bone bruise, stone bruise). Presumably, because of relative lack of soft tissue cushioning over these areas, the periosteum of the bone is contused, and periostea reactions are notoriously slow to clear. Treatment consists of appropriately placed and cut out foam rubber pads. Work on the feet may have to be restricted for a considerable period of time.

PAINFUL HEEL (*)

Although not statistically represented in this case sampling, painful heel is a fairly common complaint. It may occur following a jump from a height, landing on the heel, or in relation to some unaccustomed work on hard surfaces and so be reported as compensable injury. It is often seen in joggers and, among its many other titles, is sometimes called "jogger's heel."

Pain and tenderness occur on the bottom of the weight bearing portion of the heel at the point of insertion of the bow-string ligament of the longtiduinal arch. Symptoms tend to be most severe on first bearing weight in the morning and subside to some extent with continuing activitiy. A combination of high traction force exerted upon a small area of the periosteum of the heel by the bow-string ligament and a superimposed nonspecific inflammatory reaction seems to be the best explanation for the pain.

X-rays may show a bony spur of the calcaneus at the point of maximum tenderness and, for many years, the spur was thought to be responsible for the symptoms. As often as not, however, x-rays of the opposite normal heel will show the same type of spur, sometimes even larger than that of the symptomatic heel.

Treatment includes both mechanical and anti-inflammatory modalities. Resilient heel pads, cut out doughnut-style under the painful area, commercial plastic heel cups and longitudinal arch supports have all been used with varying degrees of success. Because of chronicity, non-steroidal anti-inflammatory medications are most commonly used and it is generally wise to prepare the patient for a long period of annoying but seldom disabling symptoms.

CHAPTER 7
THE ANKLE (60)

The ankle is a mortise and tenon joint (Figure 30). The mortise is made up of the lower tibia with its medial malleolus on the inner side and the distal fibula which terminates in the lateral malleolus on the outer side. The snugness of the mortise is maintained by the tibio-fibular ligament which binds the lower ends of the two leg bones together. The tenon is the block-like body of the talus which fits into the inverted U formed by the articular surfaces of the tibia and the two malleoli.

The ankle is supported on its inner side by the medial collateral ligament which is wide, thick and strong (Figure 31a). On the outer side support is furnished by the three-band lateral collateral ligament complex, all three bands of which are relatively thin and weak (Figure 31b). An anterior band runs forward from the tip of the lateral malleolus to anchor into the talus. A middle band runs downward to attach into the calcaneus. The posterior band runs horizontally

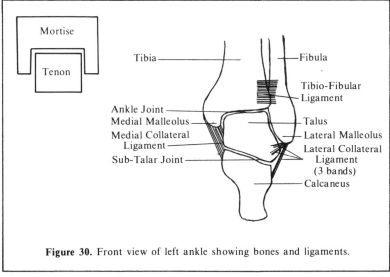

Figure 30. Front view of left ankle showing bones and ligaments.

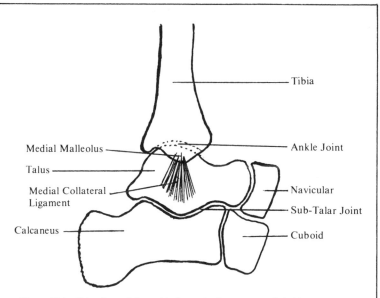

Figure 31A. Side view of the ankle from the inner or medial side.

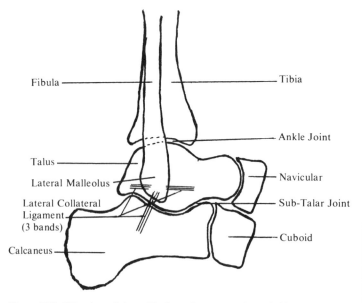

Figure 31B. Side view of the ankle from the outer or lateral side.

backward to insert into the back part of the talus.

With the exception of a very small amount of rotation, only hinge motion takes place at the ankle joint. The foot can be moved upward into dorsi-flexion about 15 degrees or downward into plantar-flexion about 45 degrees. All tilting of the foot in inversion and eversion occurs at the sub-talar joint. The other talar joints allow a limited amount of rotation of the foot, but this motion is largely blocked by the rigid sole of the average working shoe.

Most ankle injuries occur when tilting or rotational forces applied to the foot exceed the limited range of motion allowed by the tarsal joints and are transmitted through to the ankle. Inversion - internal rotation forces generally produce ankle sprains or "sprain fractures" in which the stressed ligament, instead of tearing within its substance, pulls off its attachment into bone (avulsion fracture). Eversion - external rotation forces usually produce true fractures of one or more of the malleoli and, generally, are more severe injuries.

If forces are sufficiently great, either mechanism of injury is capable of disrupting the ankle joint and, unless skillfully managed, producing high degrees of permanent disability. Fractures resulting from eversion - external rotation stress usually present an obvious threat to the integrity of the joint and are referred without hesitation to specialist care. Injuries associated with forced inversion - internal rotation are more subtle and require careful examination to identify the severe cases in which the stability of the ankle may be in jeopardy. Missing the diagnosis of a severe sprain-type injury and failing to provide the special treatment indicated leads to unstable or "trick" ankles and an almost guaranteed permanent and painful disability.

SPRAINS (43)

The common or garden-variety sprain (36) results from an inward twist of the foot combined with a variable degree of forward momentum of the body. The foot is forced into inversion, internal rotation and plantar flexion. Usually, partial tears of the anterior band and, perhaps, the middle band of the lateral collateral ligament occur, the exact distribution and degree of damage depending upon the direction and magnitude of the component forces. The point of maximum tenderness will most likely be just in front of the tip of the lateral malleolus. It is well to palpate over the other two bands of the ligament, however, to exclude damage of those components as well. Injury to the middle band produces tenderness beneath the tip of the lateral malleolus and involvement of the posterior band is associated with tenderness behind the malleolus. If the ankle is seen reasonably soon after injury, the points of tenderness are well separated and accurate determination as to which band or bands of the ligament have been injured is relatively easy. The region of the tibio-fibular ligament should also be palpated. This lies more on the anterior aspect of the ankle and an inch or more above the tip of the lateral malleolus.

Point tenderness and swelling over all three bands of the lateral collateral ligament or over the tibio-fibular ligament are warning signs that more than a common sprain has occurred and should trigger careful investigation for ankle instability.

Given evidence of a single band lateral collateral ligament sprain, initial treatment is with ice, compression and elevation until swelling has been controlled, followed by ambulation with support in the form of adhesive strapping, elastic bandage or commercial elastic cuff. Crutch or cane support may be necessary for a few days. Healing is usually complete in about three weeks and the threat of permanency is minimal.

Severe sprains (7) result from the same mechanism of injury as do simple sprains, but with greater magnitude of the component forces. There may be **complete tear of the lateral collateral ligament complex (4)** or **tear of the tibio-fibular ligament (3).** In either case, there is instability of the ankle joint. There may be indications for surgical repair. At very least, periods of rigid fixation in plaster for two to three months will be necessary.

Early recognition of the severe sprain is the key to successful management. Clinically, the severe sprain shows more swelling, more ecchymosis and presents more severe pain than does the average simple sprain. If seen early, there will be tenderness to palpation over each of the injured bands of the lateral collateral ligament or over the tibio-fibular ligament. In the severe sprain, there is often tenderness and sometimes swelling on the medial side of the ankle, as well as on the lateral side. Since this could not occur with inversion-internal rotation thrust unless joint disruption of some degree had taken place, it is a valuable, if ominous, clinical sign.

Attempt should be made, by comparing the injured with the uninjured ankle, to determine whether there is perceptible false motion, either side to side or front to back, of the foot, with relation to the leg. If muscle spasm has set in, it may not be possible to make this determination clinically. Stress x-rays should be ordered but there may be too much pain to allow proper positioning for this examination. Examination and special x-rays may have to be made under anaesthesia to determine the degree of instability.

In complete tear of the lateral collateral ligament complex (4), stress x-rays are made by taking an antero-posterior view of both ankles on the same film with the feet held in maximum inversion. Mechanical positioning devices to secure this position can be bought or made or, lacking these, the examiner may hold the feet, having first donned lead apron and gloves. Normally, the top surfaces of the talus bones will maintain a position parallel with the articular surface of the tibiae and all inversion will occur at the sub-talar joint. In severe lateral ligament sprain with ankle instability, the body of the talus of the injured ankle may tilt as much as 25 to 30 degrees into inversion (Figure 32). Since some individuals may show a few degrees of talar tilt normally, it is important that the injured ankle be compared with the opposite normal ankle.

Abnormal talar tilt is clear indication of ankle instability. In the

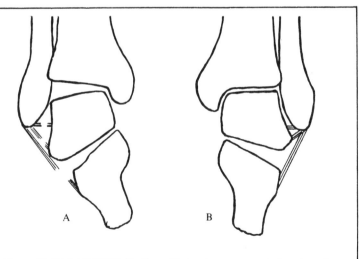

Figure 32. TALAR TILT. Outline of bones in antero-posterior view of both ankles with the feet held in maximum inversion. The injured ankle on the left (A) shows a talar tilt of about 15 degrees. All three bands of the lateral collateral ligament are torn. In the uninjured ankle (B) on the right; there is no tilt of the talus in the mortise and the lateral ligament is intact. All inversion motion is occurring at the sub-talar joint.

young high-caliber athlete, surgical repair is sometimes done. For most patients, swelling is controlled by the usual methods and the ankle is immobilized in a walking plaster boot for about eight weeks.

In tibio-fibular ligament tear (3), the point of maximum tenderness is well above the lateral malleolus and more anterior. Instability may be easier to detect, clinically, than in the complete lateral ligament tear. On x-ray examination, antero-posterior views of both ankles may show a widening of the ankle mortise on the injured side (Figure 33). Normally, the space between the medial border of the talus and the inner surface of the medial malleolus should be the same as that between the top of the talus and the articular surface of the tibia. With a spread mortise, the medial space is widened and this can readily be noted when compared with the opposite ankle.

Certain cases of spread mortise may be considered for surgery. It is usually necessary to draw the tibia and fibula together with lag screws or bolts and nuts to reconstitute the mortise. The tibio-fibular ligament is repaired and the hardware removed when healing is complete. Milder cases are treated in plaster casts with compression applied to the well-padded malleoli as the cast is setting. Frequently, neither method is entirely successful and some degree of permanency is likely.

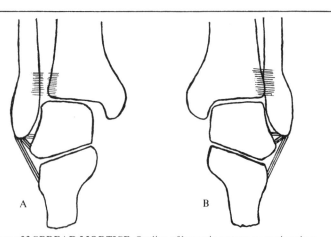

Figure 33 SPREAD MORTISE. Outline of bones in antero-posterior view of both ankles. The injured ankle (A) on the left shows spread of the ankle mortise. The distance between the medial cortex of the talus and the inner side of the medial malleolus is greater than the distance between the top surface of the talus and the articular surface of the tibia. The tibio-fibular ligament is torn. The normal ankle (B) on the right shows normal relationships at the ankle joint.

FRACTURES (13)

Fractures about the ankle can be most clearly presented and understood according to the mechanism of injury. Those resulting from inversion and internal rotation forces are quite different and ordinarily much less threatening than those which occur with eversion and external rotation.

Inversion-Internal Rotation Fractures (7)

Avulsion fracture of the tip of the fibula (6) results from the sprain mechanism of injury but, instead of a tear of the ligament, the bony insertion of the lateral ligament into the tip of the lateral malleolus is avulsed. The fractures are generally small chips and the fracture lines are transverse and close to the tip of the malleolus. The x-ray appearance (Figure 34A) is quite different from that of fractures of the lower end of the fibula associated with eversion - external rotation injury which will be discussed later.

Treatment is determined by the presence or absence of instability of the ankle joint. If there is no instability, avulsion fractures of the tip of the fibula are treated like simple sprains. If ankle instability is present or suspected, immobilization in a plaster boot is indicated as in severe sprain.

Inversion fracture of the tibia (1) is usually associated with strong upward compression of the ankle with the foot inverted, as in jumping and landing on an incline. The talus is tilted sufficiently in the mortise to act as a wedge to split off the lower tibia from the base of the medial malleolus obliquely upward (Figure 34B). There often is no displacement, but the presence of this type of fracture is evidence of joint disruption and mandates cast immobilization as for severe sprain. Displaced fractures will often require open reduction and fixation.

Eversion-External Rotation Fractures (6)

These fractures are potentially more threatening to the architecture and stability of the ankle joint. They exhibit an interesting progression in severity (Figure 35) depending upon the magnitude of the injuring force.

Spiral fracture of the distal fibula (3) is the first stage of this progression

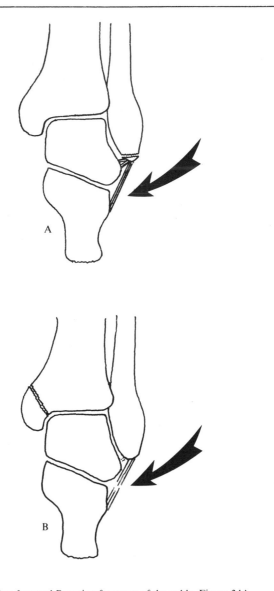

Figure 34. Inversion-Internal Rotation fractures of the ankle. Figure 34A
shows the typical avulsion fracture of the tip of the fibula, the bony
attachment of the lateral ligament having been torn off. Figure 34B shows
an inversion fracture of the tibia. The talus, tilting in the mortise, acts as a
wedge to split off the medial malleolus obliquely.

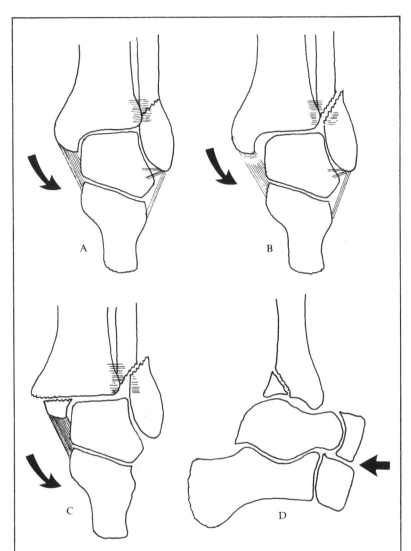

Figure 35. Progression of severity in eversion - external rotation fractures of the ankle. In 35A, a spiral oblique fracture of the fibula has occurred without displacement, leaving the ligaments intact. In 35B, there is lateral displacement of the distal fibula and of the talus. Either the medial collateral ligament or the tibio-fibular ligament or both must be ruptured. Ankle is unstable. In 35C, the talus has shifted laterally and the medial collateral ligament has pulled off the medial malleolus (bi-malleolar fracture). In 35D, both malleoli have fractured and the talus is posteriorly displaced, knocking off the posterior lip of the tibia (tri-malleolar fracture).

(Figure 35A). As the foot is forced into external rotation and eversion, the talus is externally rotated in the ankle mortise, the strong medial ligament holds as a pivot point, and the lower end of the fibula fractures in a spiral oblique pattern. The spiral extends upward from the surface of the fibula facing the tibia and it may originate below, above, or at the level of the tibio-fibular ligament. If there is no displacement, these fractures can usually be treated in a plaster boot. A walking device may be added to the boot after a week or two and healing is usually complete in about six weeks.

If the fracture is displaced (Figure 35B), there is a clear signal that further damage has occurred somewhere in the ankle joint. Either there is an unseen fracture of the medial malleolus, the medial collateral ligament has torn, or there is a tear of the tibio-fibular ligament. It is best to refer all patients with displaced spiral oblique fractures of the distal fibula for specialist care. Joint integrity is at risk.

Bi-malleolar fractures (2) represent progression of the injury mechanism after the distal fibular has fractured. The talus is forced laterally and the strong medial collateral ligament avulses the medial malleolus, usually by a transverse fracture across its base (Figure 35C). The degree of displacement may vary from minimal all the way to severe lateral subluxation of the ankle joint.

Specialist care is required. Exact anatomical reduction of both malleoli and restoration of the ankle mortise must be achieved. Open reduction is frequently necessary.

Tri-malleolar fracture (1) is the end stage of the injury progression and represents a true fracture-dislocation of the ankle. Having fractured both malleoli, the talus is locked in external rotation and the foreward momentum of the body pushes the tibia forward and fractures its posterior lip, which is sometimes called the third malleolus (Figure 35D). The fracture usually extends obliquely upward and may involve a significant portion of the aricular surface of the tibia. Specialist care is required and the entire ankle must be reconstructed, usually by open reduction and internal fixation.

In all severe ankle injuries requiring specialist care, speed in the delivery of the patient to the definitive treatment facility is highly important. Swelling occurs rapidly in these injuries and the bony landmarks which are so helpful in attempted closed reductions are soon obliterated. Fracture blebs and blisters may appear within hours and so compromise the viability and integrity of the skin as to force delay in open procedures.

Ice, compression and elevation should be quickly applied, a splint arranged for transportation and the patient evacuated at once. Commercial inflatable plastic splints are available in most dispensaries. Lacking that, a pillow can be firmly bound to the foot and lower leg as a splint. The badly injured ankle ranks high on the list of true medical emergencies.

CONTUSIONS (4)

Contusions about the ankle deserve mention because they often break the thin skin overlying the malleoli, are prone to infection, and heal slowly because of the relatively slow circulation in the area. Especially in older patients or in those with varicose veins, the contusions must be thoroughly cleansed, the dressings changed frequently and the circulation in the lower leg supported by elastic stockings or bandages.

CHAPTER 8
THE KNEE (72)

Judged as an articulating device between two long weight-bearing bones, capable of 135 degrees of hinge motion, but inherently resistant to powerful angulating and rotational stresses, the knee would win few awards for excellent of engineering design.

The bony contours of the lower end of the femur and the upper end of the tibia provide virtually no architectural stability for the joint. The lower femur terminates in two rounded condyles, somewhat similar to the humeral condyles at the elbow. The upper tibia, however, has only two flat surfaces, the tibial plateaus, upon which the femoral condyles rest and move (Figure 36). There is nothing in the shape of the bones to prevent sideways wobble of the hinge nor front to back sliding of the femur on the tibia.

The flat tibial plateaus are converted into shallow cups for better contouring with the rounded femoral condyles by the addition of the medial and lateral menisci (Figure 37). A meniscus is somewhat like a tapered half-washer attached to the peripheral margin of each plateau. Made of dense fibro-cartilage, the meniscus is wedge-shaped in cross section, the base of the wedge conforming to the outer margins of the plateau and the apex facing inward toward the center of the joint. Except for a narrow peripheral margin where they are attached, the menisci have no blood supply and are therefore incapable of healing when torn or damaged. In normal hinge motion, they bear little or no weight and serve only to fill the space between the flat plateau and the rounded condyle. When the knee is subjected to rotational stress, however, the femoral condyles may ride up onto the menisci, and tearing and shredding can result.

The knee is stabilized to some degree against sideways wobble by medial and lateral ligaments (Figure 38). The medial ligament is the stronger and clinically more important of the two since most sideways injuring forces approach from the outer side of the knee. It is composed of two layers: a deep band bridges the short span from joint margin to joint margin, and a more superficial, triangular-shaped layer attaches

97

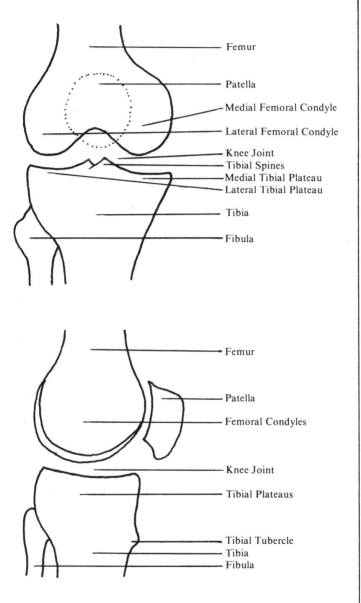

Figure 36. Bony landmarks of the knee. Above is a front view of the right knee. Below is a side view from the medial side of the knee. The contour of the bones provides no architectural stability for the joint.

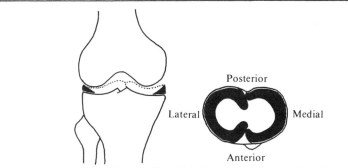

Figure 37. The menisci. The flat tibial plateaus are converted into shallow cups by the addition of tapered half-washers, one for the medial, one for the lateral plateau. Seen in cross section on the left, they are wedge-shaped, tapering into the interior of the joint. On the right is a view of the medial and lateral menisci looking downward onto the tibial plateaus.

by its apex to the femoral condyle an inch or so above the joint and by its base to a broad area along the inner side of the tibia an inch or so below the joint. Since the superficial layer is apt to be torn first in knee sprains and since the tear is most likely to occur near one or the other of its bony attachments, points of maximum tenderness in mild or moderate knee sprains usually occur away from the joint line and provide valuable clinical clues in the differential diagnosis of the common injuries to the medial side of the knee. The lateral ligament, extending from the lateral epicondyle of the femur to the head of the fibula, is rarely injured.

Forward and backward sliding of the femur on the tibia is controlled by a pair of short ligaments, the cruciates, which lie deep in the center of the joint and criss-cross the space between the inner bony surfaces of the femoral condyles and two bony prominences, the tibial spines, which lie between the tibial plateaus (Figure 38). Taking their designations from their lower attachments into the tibia, the anterior cruciate ligament crosses from the anterior tibial spine backward, laterally and upwards to the back of the lateral femoral condyle and keeps the femur from sliding backward on the tibia. The posterior cruciate ligaments crosses from the posterior tibial spine forward, medially and upwards to the front of the medial femoral condyle and prevents the femur from sliding forward on the tibia.

In addition to their function in checking fore and aft sliding of the femur on the tibia, their direction gives them some ability to control sideways wobble. In a severe knee sprain, laterally approaching force may tear, first the superficial layer of the medial ligament, then the deep

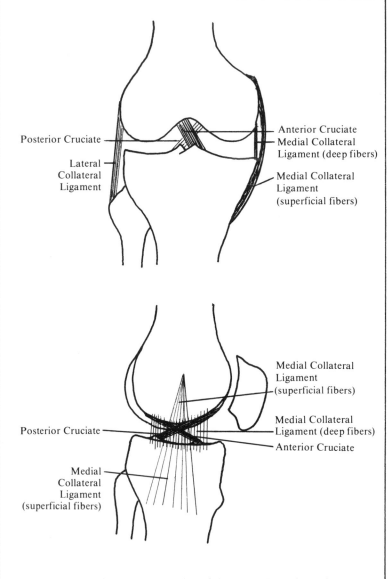

Figure 38. The ligaments. Front view of right knee above shows the two layers of the medial ligament, the lateral ligament and, in the center of the joint, the cruciate ligaments. Side view of inner side of knee shows the deltoid shape of the superficial fibers of the medial ligament with the broad base of insertion into the tibia.

layer, and finally, the anterior cruciate ligament. The cruciates may also be stressed and damaged by rotational forces applied to the knee.

In view of the potential magnitude of the deforming forces and the long lever arms through which they are exerted, the ligament support system is inadequate, and the knee is heavily dependent upon the muscles of the thigh for support.

The most important of these is the quadriceps, a complex of four muscles which make up the contour of the front of the thigh. Their tendon fibers converge to attach along the upper edge of the patella and their pull is transmitted to the tibia by fibers arising from the lower edge of the patella and inserting into the tibial tubercle (Figure 36). In effect, the patella is incorporated in the quadriceps tendon and serves to increase the mechanical advantage of the quadriceps muscle in delivering forceful extension of the knee.

Viewed in cross section, the underside of the patella is V shaped and the V fits into the groove between the two femoral condyles keeping the powerful pull of the quadriceps on track. The posterior surface of the patella is covered by articular cartilage for smooth upward and downward gliding against the underlying femoral condyles during the hinge motion of the knee. While anatomically separate from the true knee joint, the patello-femoral joint plays an important role in knee function and is subject to its own group of injuries, dysfunctions and important clinical conditions.

The patello-femoral joint lies in an extension of the snyovial lined capsule of the knee joint called the supra-patellar pouch which reaches a full hand's-breadth above the superior margin of the patella. This pouch participates in effusions of the knee and provides the safest area in which to aspirate the knee joint. An aspirating needle usually is inserted into the pouch about an inch above and lateral to the patella and the knee joint can thus be tapped without danger of damage by the point of the needle to the main femoral or tibial articular cartilage.

The articular cartilage on the back of the knee cap is damaged in virtually every fracture of the patella. Blows to the front of the knee which do not fracture the patella may also inflict damage upon this cartilage layer as the patella is rammed back against the underlying bone of the femoral condyles. A bruise of the articular cartilage may cause a hollowed-out, degenerated area since cartilage has but little power of healing. This degeneration is known as chondromalacia patellae and may cause pain, audible snaps and cracks, feelings of instability, and even locking sensations in the knee as the pitted area in the surface of the back of the patella is drawn forcibly over the convexity of the femoral condyle with the compression force resulting from quadriceps contraction.

The hamstring muscles in the back of the thigh contribute materially to the support of the knee. The medial hamstring, especially, offers backup to the medial and cruciate ligaments since its lower tendon attaches over a broad surface on the inner and front surfaces of the tibia.

Preservation and restoration of the mass and power of the thigh muscles, especially the quadriceps, is the keynote to the successful management of knee injuries. Significant degrees of ligamentous laxity can be compensated for by strong thigh muscles, allowing essentially normal knee function. On the other hand, an architecturally perfect knee with normal ligaments can be painful and unstable if activity is allowed before full thigh muscle power has been regained.

In athletics, the knee is the most vulnerable joint in the body. In this sampling of cases, the knee ranks only behind the hand and foot in incidence of extremity injuries and carries a higher risk of permanent disability than either.

The knee area is equipped with a number of bursae which may cause clinical problems. Most commonly involved are those that protect the bony prominences on the front of the knee, the patella and the tibial tubercle, from external friction and irritation such as may occur in kneeling work. A bursa is situated between the superficial and deep layers of the medial ligament. The deep layer of the ligament, bridging from articular margin to articular margin, is relatively fixed. The superficial layer, however, traverses as the joint moves from flexion to extension and the bursa is inserted to prevent friction between the two layers. A bursa-like structure is located over the posterior surface of the knee in the region of the medial hamstring tendon, and often communicates with the joint. When distended, this structure is known as a Baker's cyst.

As in the eversion-external rotation injuries of the ankle, there is a progression pattern in the soft tissue injuries to the vulnerable medial aspect of the knee. Most injury forces approach from the outer side, catching the knee weight bearing, in a position of slight flexion and with varying degrees of external rotation of the foot. As the knee is forced into knock-knee position, a sequence of injury is initiated, the extent of progression dependent upon the severity and duration of the injuring force. Evaluation of the sprained knee can be more intelligently carried out if this sequence is carried in mind.

PROGRESSION OF INJURY TO THE MEDIAL SIDE OF THE KNEE

1. Stretching or tearing of the superficial fibers of the medial ligament (mild sprain)
   a. Tenderness above or below the joint line
   b. Soft tissue swelling in area of tenderness
   c. No effusion in joint
   d. No medio-lateral instability

2. The above plus stretching or tearing of the deep fibers of the medial ligament (moderate or severe sprain)
   a. Tenderness above or below and at the joint line
   b. Soft tissue swelling diffuse over medial side of knee
   c. May be effusion in the joint
   d. Medio-lateral instability, moderate (up to 15 degrees) or severe (more than 15 degrees)

3. All the above plus stretching or tearing of the anterior cruciate ligament
   a. Diffuse tenderness over entire medial side of knee
   b. Marked swelling over medial side of knee
   c. Effusion in the joint
   d. Medio-lateral instability, usually severe
   e. Antero-posterior instability (tibia can be pulled forward on femur = positive drawer sign)

4. All the above plus tear of the medial meniscus
   a. Diffuse swelling and tenderness medially and anteriorly
   b. Effusion in the joint
   c. Medio-lateral and antero-posterior instability
   d. Tenderness over meniscus (halfway between mid-anterior and mid-medial planes on the joint line)
   e. May be block to full extension of the knee

Table 3. Progression of medial side knee injuries.

SPRAINS (27)

Medial Ligament (25)

Medial ligament sprains may result from forced external rotation of the tibia on the femur, as in the typical ski injury, or from direct lateral force to the outer side of the knee, as in blocking in football, or from a combination of these two mechanisms. As in all sprains, the first task is to assess the degree of instability, if any, of the joint. Knees, more than most joints, vary from person to person in the degree of lateral laxity normally present and the normal knee must be carefully evaluated before the injured knee is approached. Lateral wobble is tested with the knee flexed 30 degrees from the fully extended position with the patient supine and relaxed on the examining table. Inward pressure is exerted with one hand on the outer side of the thigh while the other hand pulls the lower leg into the knock-knee position.

In mild sprain, the point of maximum tenderness is usually over one of the other attachment of the superficial fibers of the ligament, about an inch above or below the joint line. There will be little or no tenderness on the joint line, itself, and no detectable lateral instability. Stressing the joint into the knock-knee position will cause pain accurately referred to the point of maximum tenderness.

In mild sprains without instability, an elastic bandage wrap over a felt popliteal pad is usually sufficient support. Crutches may be necessary for the first few days. Healing time is usually about three weeks. Quadriceps exercises should be started at once, usually beginning with straight leg lifts or isometric exercises that will not demand motion of the knee. Knee extension exercises are instituted as soon as they can be tolerated by the patient and no patient is allowed to return to full activity, particularly athletic participation, until strength testing and thigh circumference measurements indicate full recovery of quadriceps mass and power.

Moderate sprains may show tenderness at joint level in addition to the points of tenderness over the upper or lower attachments of the superficial portion of the ligament and there may be detectable instability. These injuries should be more rigidly immobilized, usually in a plaster walking cylinder, for a longer period of time, commonly six to eight weeks. Quadriceps exercises must, of necessity, be limited to straight leg lifts and isometrics while the cast is in place, but, on removal of the cast, a formal routine of heavy resistance exercises should be instituted and, again, the patient must demonstrate full recovery of thigh muscle power and mass before being allowed to return to full activity. Undue reliance should not be placed on the typical commercial elastic knee cuff as a protector of the knee during this recovery period. On the average, it will take about the same length of time out of plaster as the patient was in the plaster cylinder to recover full muscle power and adequate protection of the knee.

In severe sprains with marked instability, surgical repair of the ligament should be considered, depending upon the age and activity level of the patient. Specialist opinion is indicated.

Lateral Ligament (1)

Not a common injury, lateral ligament sprains are managed by the same rules as pertain to medial ligament sprains. They generally carry less threat of permanency and seldom produce significant instability of the joint.

Cruciate ligament (1)

Rarely, impact directly to the front or to the back of the knee area may produce an isolated sprain of either the anterior or the posterior cruciate ligament. Again, the key to treatment is the degree of instability of the joint. Antero-posterior instability is best tested in the sitting position with the patient's legs flexed 90 degrees over the edge of the examining table. The tibia is pulled forward upon the femur to evaluate anterior cruciate laxity and pushed backward toward the table edge to assess posterior cruciate laxity. The tibial plateau area is easily seen and false motion of it in relation to the femoral condyles can usually be observed if there is instability. As is the case with the medial and lateral ligaments, there is a wide range of normal for cruciate ligament snugness and no judgement can be made on the injured knee until the well knee has been carefully evaluated. Any degree of detectable antero-posterior instability of the tibia upon the femur is grounds for referral for expert opinion since the chances of other damage within the joint are good. Cruciate ligament sprains without instability can be treated as outlined for mild medial ligament sprains.

TEAR OF MENISCUS (20)

Isolated tears of the menisci are relatively uncommon. Usually, some other damage to ligaments is necessary to allow sufficient rotation of the femoral condyles to ride up onto and tear a meniscus. Since most ligamentous damage occurs on the medial side of the knee, it is the medial meniscus which is most frequently torn (19). When a lateral meniscus is torn (1), there is a good chance that it was an abnormally shaped meniscus from birth. Congenital discoid lateral meniscus is the common abnormality and, in this condition, the lateral meniscus is very broad, often nearly covering the entire lateral tibial plateau.

Medial meniscus tears usually result from rotational force. In one typical mechanism of injury in football, the ball carrier is running parallel to the line of scrimmage, spots a hole and plants the right foot preparatory to cutting to the left into the hole. With the extreme internal rotation of the femur upon the fixed tibia and with the knee semi-flexed and bearing full weight, the right knee collapses and the player falls to the ground, often without any contact by an opposing player. The medial femoral condyle has ridden up onto the medial meniscus and torn the cartilage, often by splitting its circumferential fibers, producing the "bucket-handle" tear of the medial meniscus. The split-off inner portion of the meniscus may then deflect into the inner portion of the joint, attached only at its front and back mooring points, and lock the knee, making full extension impossible.

Having witnessed or listened to the description of the injury, and faced with a locked knee and effusion in the joint, there is little difficulty in making the diagnosis. Most cases, however, are not so clear cut and a tear of the meniscus may be only one of several features of the progression of injury to the medial side of the knee. The meniscus may not tear in classical "bucket-handle" fashion. Often, there are tears of the anterior or posterior attachments, or partial tears of the inner margins.

Clinically, there is usually effusion in the knee joint. The point of maximum tenderness is on the medial joint line about halfway between the mid anterior and mid medial planes. There may be a firm block to full extension of the knee, but this sign must be interpretted cautiously since effusion or hamstring spasm will also make full extension of the knee difficult or impossible. Since there is likely to be some element of ligamentous damage as well, tenderness along the medial side of the joint is often diffuse over the medial ligament as well as at the typical meniscus point. Pain and effusion may make stress testing for ligamentous damage virtually impossible without anaesthesia. Any knee showing effusion in the joint within a short time after injury involving torsional or lateral stress while weight-bearing deserves early referral to a specialist. Arthrography and arthroscopy are increasingly accurate diagnostic procedures and, in isolated meniscus injuries, arthroscopic surgery is materially shortening the period of disability.

A somewhat unusual mechanism of meniscus tear is seen occasionally in the workplace. Because the two femoral condyles have slightly different radii and centers of arc, the hinge motion of the knee is accompanied by a small amount of rotatory motion of tibia upon femur as the joint hinges from full extension to full flexion. In full extension, the tibia is rotated about 15 degrees into internal rotation relative to the femur. In full flexion, there is about 15 degrees of external rotation of tibia upon femur. Occasionally, following a period of time working in the full knee-flexed position, sitting on the heels, sudden resumption of the upright position will cause the medial femoral condyle, which has ridden up onto the back surface of the medial meniscus during the period of full flexion, to ride along the medial meniscus and cause a split in its fibers as the knee is rapidly extended. A true "bucket-handle" tear of the meniscus may result. The diagnosis may not even be entertained because of the seeming lack of significant injury. Meniscal tears by this mechanism are seen in roofers, flooring and carpet installers and service people working on machinery close to the floor.

Because of the lack of blood supply except at the very margins of attachment, most meniscal tears do not heal. Minor tears may cause relatively little disability, but they often produce recurrent symptoms on pivoting motions and the patient is said to have a "trick knee". If the frequency of recurrent episodes becomes disabling or the unreliability of the knee becomes dangerous, such patients should be referred for surgical resection of the meniscus. Following meniscus surgery, patients are able to undertake full normal activity, including athletics, but studies indicate that the operated knees show degenerative arthritic changes earlier than do normal knees.

CONTUSIONS (8)

A direct blow to the front of the knee, as in a forward fall landing on the hands and knees, is often followed by bleeding into the joint. Effusion usually appears within an hour or so and may distend the joint capsule so tightly as to produce severe pain. If so, the joint can be aspirated and the blood withdrawn. There is a statistical danger of infection associated with aspiration, however, and most post-traumatic effusions are treated by ice packs and compression.

Fractures of the patella must be excluded by x-ray in such injuries. As in all knee injuries, quadriceps exercises must be started at once. Straight leg lifts can generally be done without too much discomfort, but knee motion exercises must be deferred until the effusion has subsided.

BURSITIS (8)

Pre-Patellar Bursitis (6)

Commonly known as housemaid's knee, even though there are few housemaids and scrubbing floors on the hands and knees is all but unheard of, pre-patellar bursitis is still seen among kneeling workers. In the same area, and affected by the same activities, are two other anterior bursae, one over the tibial tubercle and one over the patellar tendon.

Treatment usually includes aspiration of the bursa with injection of steroids and provision of a protective pad along with proscription of kneeling work. Rarely, the bursal swelling becomes chronic with thickening of the bursal walls and recurrent effusions and surgical excision may become necessary. Occasionally, infection develops in a pre-patellar bursa and become a serious problem. Rigid sterile precautions should be observed whenever aspiration of bursae along the front of the knee is undertaken.

Medial Collateral Ligament Bursitis (1)

Irritation of the bursa between the deep and superficial layers of the medial ligament may occur after activity involving repeated squatting and standing. Swelling of the bursa is not readily apparent, since it lies just beneath the leading edge of the superficial layer of the ligament. With the knee flexed, it can sometimes be felt as a small, firm, tender nodule. As the knee extends, it retracts beneath the ligament. Pain, which may be severe, is aggravated by direct pressure, as in sleeping on the side with the knees together, and by sudden external rotation of the foot. The point of tenderness is very close to that found in tear of the medial meniscus, and diagnostic confusion may arise. Treatment is by local injection of a steroid, most easily performed with the knee in flexion.

Baker's Cyst (1)

The appearance of a painful cystic swelling in the back of the knee over the medial hamstring tendon after activity such as working on a ladder which involves hyper-extension of the knee suggests Baker's cyst. A high percentage of such cysts communicate with the knee joint and may indicate abnormality in the posterior compartment, often in the region of posterior attachment of the medial meniscus. If modification of activity or aspiration and injection with steroids fail to relieve the condition, referral to a specialist is probably wise. An arthrogram may be necessary to exclude intra-articular abnormality in the posterior compartment of the knee.

CHONDROMALACIA PATELLAE (6)

Roughening of the posterior cartilaginous surface of the patella can produce pain and a feeling of instability in the knee, as well as being responsible for considerable creaking and cracking of the joint. The function of the patella as a sort of fulcrum over which the quadriceps muscle exerts its force in straightening the knee means that its posterior surface is pressed hard against the rather sharp convexity of the underlying femoral condyles, especially when the knee is extended against heavy resistance, as in stair or ladder climbing. Any irregularity of the cartilage surface is likely to be irritated as it is scrubbed against the opposing surface of the condyle.

Some cases of chondromalacia occur after a single injury. A direct blow to the front of the knee, not quite hard enough to produce fracture of the patella, may cause a bruise of the cartilage on the back of the knee cap. Because of the poor healing qualities of cartilage, a dimple of softened and degenerated cartilage may develop at the site of the bruise and cause pain each time it passes over the convexity of the condyle.

Chondromalacia more often occurs as an attritional change in knees in which there is mal-alignment or an abnormality of bony structure affecting the contour of the femoral condyles or the shape or placement of the patella. In bow-leg or knock-knee, the pull of the quadriceps muscle through the patella to the tibial tubercle is at an angle and one side or the other of the V-shaped back surface of the patella receives increased pressure and friction as it rubs against the side of the intercondylar groove. Early degeneration of cartilage of the posterior patellar surface on that side is likely.

One or the other femoral condyle may have congenital flattening so that the groove is not well defined and the patella may actually ride into and out of the mal-formed groove as the knee is flexed and extended. Flattening of the lateral femoral condyle plus knock-knee plus poor quadriceps tone is a combination which may lead to recurrent lateral subluxation or dislocation of the patella.

Occasionally, the patella is placed abnormally high (patella alta) or low (patella baja), the fit of the patella in the intercondylar groove is poor, and abnormal friction creates degeneration of the cartilage.

Whatever the cause, patients have pain in the front of the knee, aggravated by stair climbing and by full flexion of the knees. When the condition is severe, there may be effusion in the knee joint due to a secondary synovitis. On examination, there is pain as the knee is flexed and extended while downward pressure is maintained on the knee cap. If enough relaxation can be obtained for adequate palpation, there is often localized tenderness beneath the medial border of the patella. The patient may show bow-leg, knock-knee, high or low riding patella or abnormal lateral mobility of the patella.

Treatment consists of maintenance of the fully extended position of the knee, thus avoiding pressure on the patella, by various means and for varying periods until irritation has subsided. If there is secondary synovitis, anti-inflammatory medications may be indicated. Depending upon the severity of symptoms and the ability of the patient to cooperate, avoidance of knee-flexed positions and stair climbing may be sufficient to relieve symptoms. Various reminders against knee flexion all the way from a strip of adhesive tape to pull on the skin when the knee is bent to a plaster cylinder have been used. Often, habits of sitting with the feet hooked back onto the chair or stool while at work are discovered and, if the habit can be broken, symptoms may disappear.

Rarely, chondromalacia patellae is sufficiently severe so that surgical smoothing of the back surface of the patella or even resection of the patella may have to be considered.

TRAUMATIC SYNOVITIS (3)

Secondary inflammation of the synovial lining of the joint may follow contusion, sprain, meniscus injury or chrondromalacia patellae and the diagnosis should really be that of the precipitating injury. If the synovitis is persistent after the effects of the initiating trauma have cleared, it may have to be treated by anti-inflammatory drugs, either systemically or locally.

If injury seems doubtful or inadequate to produce the degree of synovial reaction and effusion present, arthritis and gout should be considered. Aspiration of the joint with full chemical and microscopic study of the synovial fluid may be necessary for diagnosis.

FRACTURES (*)

Although not statistically represented in this sampling of 1,000 cases, fractures about the knee obviously do occur in the working population. They almost always require specialist care, often for open procedures.

Patella (*)

Only minor chip fractures and certain undisplaced incomplete fractures can be managed on an ambulatory basis. Most patellar fractures are comminuted and, because of the pull of the quadriceps, widely displaced. Treatment is surgical. If, under direct vision, the fragments cannot be reduced so as to produce a smooth articulating posterior surface, patellectomy may be necessary. Providing the lateral expansions of the quadriceps tendon are firmly sutured and the central tendon is reefed and over-lapped to make up for the length of the missing patella, the functional results are often quite good.

Tibial Plateau (*)

As the result of a fall from a height, landing on the feet, the flat tibial plateau may be driven upward against the rounded femoral condyle with sufficient force to produce fractures somewhat like those which occur in the head of the radius at the elbow. The plateau may be split and part or all of it depressed. The entire plateau may be shattered and the fragments driven down into the tibial shaft. Surgical treatment is necessary if there is any degree of displacement and if there has been extensive comminution and impaction, the prognosis must be guarded. If adequate restoration of plateau height and smoothness of articular surface cannot be achieved, metallic or plastic plateau prostheses may have to be used.

CHAPTER 9
THE LEG (20)

Exclude the joints with their intricacies of design and function and their broad range of pathomechanical responses to injury and attrition, and the remainder of the leg loses much of its interest, at least as the site of orthopaedic problems amenable to dispensary care. The long bones are subject to fracture, but mainly in obvious and major accidents, and their treatment nearly always requires hospitalization and specialist care. Leg muscles occasionally fail to meet demands for powerful thrust and ruptures, partial or complete, of muscle or tendon constitute the chief area of concern to occupational physicians and nurses.

FRACTURES (7)

Femur (2)

Femoral shaft fractures involve only diagnosis and preparation for transfer for definitive care. The Thomas splint is still the safest and most comfortable transport device. If none is available, the injured leg can often be bound to the well leg or a long board extending from under the arm to beyond the foot can be used as a splint.

If femoral shaft fractures are compound, a dry sterile dressing should be applied to the compound wound and no attempt should be made to improve the position of the fragments and thus risk sucking contaminated bone ends back under the skin.

Tibia and fibula (2)

Fractures of the shafts of both bones of the lower leg, like those of the femur, require only diagnosis and evacuation. A Thomas splint, a full-length plastic inflatable splint, or even a pillow splint are generally satisfactory temporary immobilization devices. The same rule applies to compound fractures as was cited for the femur.

Neck and upper shaft of fibula (3)

These are sometimes hidden fractures, caused by rotational stress, and occurring in conjunction with manifest ankle injuries. A routine clinical check for tenderness over the upper part of the fibula should be made as part of the examination in every ankle sprain. The peroneal nerve winds around the neck of the fibula and is sometimes involved in fractures at that level. Foot drop can result from peroneal nerve injury and its appearance following the treatment of what apparently was a simple sprain of the ankle can be a source of embarrassment, not to mention legal problems.

Most isolated fibular shaft fractures can be treated without plaster immobilization. They are inherently stable, as a rule, due to the splinting action of the intact tibia.

Stress Fractures (*)

Stress, fatigue or insufficiency fractures, similar to the march fracture of the metatarsal neck, may occasionally occur in the leg bones and present difficulties in diagnosis. The lower end of the fibula, the mid shaft of the tibia and the neck of the femur are the most common sites.

The lower end of the fibula is a fairly frequent site for stress fracture in runners, particularly if they have recently increased the distance or speed of the run. The shaft of the tibia may be involved in athletes, usually early season or after participation in some new kind of sport. It may be mistaken for shin splints. The neck of the femur is a relatively common location for insufficiency fracture in the elderly, and it is probably true that many older people break their hip and then fall, rather than falling and breaking their hip. The occurrence of insufficiency fracture of the neck of the femur among young, active adults, however, is less well recognized and may be missed if the possibility of its occurrence is not kept in mind.

Usually, there is a history of some unusual or unaccustomed activity followed by pain over the involved bone. Examination will usually show well localized tenderness over bone, but little in the way of swelling or discoloration. X-rays will usually be negative for the first two or three weeks, but repeat examination after that interval will show a hairline crack and subsequent films will often show a massive collection of fresh bony callus. The exuberance of callus production has been mistaken for bone tumor.

MUSCLE AND TENDON RUPTURES (9)

Medial Head of Gastrocnemius (8)

A relatively common injury among middle-aged athletes, the diagnosis can almost be made by the history. With a sudden push-off motion from the weight-bearing foot, the patient experiences sharp pain in the back of the calf and, almost automatically, looks about to discover the source of external impact. Older textbooks describe the condition as rupture of the plantaris muscle, a pencil-thin muscle band which arises from the lateral femoral condyle, courses down the back of the calf and inserts into the tendo achilles. Most authorities now agree that, in most cases, it is the medial head of the gastrocnemius which ruptures partially, usually about four inches below the knee.

The patient has severe pain on attempting to raise the heel from the ground and there is well localized tenderness over the inner belly of the calf muscle a hand's breadth below the knee. If the patient is seen early, a defect in the muscle belly can often be felt. Hemorrhage may be significant and, in the days following injury, massive ecchymosis of the lower leg, ankle and foot may develop and, unless forewarned, constitute a considerable source of worry to the patient.

A heel elevation to take the pull off the gastrocnemius during the healing period is the mainstay in treatment. Crutches may be necessary for the first few days. An elastic bandage wrap of the entire lower leg, ankle and foot contributes comfort and may check the hemorrhagic ooze to some extent. There seldom is significant permanency although symptoms may persist for six to eight weeks and recurrent ruptures on the same or opposite side are not unknown.

Tendo Achilles Rupture (1)

The chief responsibility of the occupational physician or nurse is to make the diagnosis, since surgical repair is usually indicated. Diagnosis may present some difficulty, especially if the patient is not seen soon after the incident. The degree of trauma is often not impressive, either to the patient or to the examiner. The patient is able actively to plantar-flex the foot, using the peroneal muscles and the toe flexors, but usually not with sufficient power to raise body weight on tip-toe. The defect in the tendon can be palpated during the early minutes after injury, but massive swelling develops in the area within a few hours and makes this impossible.

A special test may be helpful in reaching a diagnosis. The patient sits on the examining table with both legs dangling free over the side. The calf muscle of the uninjured leg is squeezed and the foot will be noted to plantar flex. On the injured side, if the tendo achilles has been ruptured, squeezing of the calf will produce no motion of the foot.

When the diagnosis is made, the patient should be referred for specialist care at once since early surgical repair is likely to produce the best results.

CONTUSIONS (3)

Contusions of calf and thigh muscles are treated by the immediate application of cold, compression and elevation in an effort to control the deep and often extensive hemorrhage which follows. The disability may be significant and crutches may be required for several days. Support in the form of an elastic bandage wrap or elastic stocking often gives comfort and allows earlier ambulation.

Heat and massage are avoided, especially over contused thigh muscles, because of the danger of ossified hematoma (myositis ossificans). This is a real threat, particularly in the young athlete.

TENOSYNOVITIS (1)

Tenosynovitis involving the tendons about the ankle is occasionally seen. The peroneal tendons in the region of the lateral malleolus, the anterior tibial tendon at the front of the ankle, or the tendo achilles are most likely to be affected. Treatment includes the use of anti-inflammatory medications and some form of mechanical support of the ankle and foot. This may be by adhesive strapping, elastic bandage wrap or a plaster boot depending upon the degrees and severity of involvement.

Local injection of these tendons with steroids should be approached with extreme caution because of the danger of delayed tendon rupture following repeated steroid injection.

SHIN SPLINTS (*)

Not encountered in this tabulation as a compensable injury, shin splints is a fairly frequent complaint among workers. Typically seen in athletes after unaccustomed play on hard surfaces, especially in games involving start-and-stop running and frequent jumping, it may also occur in the early season runner or jogger who works out on hard surfaces.

Mild cases probably represent strain of the anterior calf muscles. These muscles are encased in a rigid compartment along the antero-lateral side of the calf. The rigid tibia and fibula with their inter-connecting fibrous tissue comprise the floor and sides of the compart-ment, and the roof is formed by a dense, firm layer of fascia. Any swelling of muscles within the compartment increases the pressure, sometimes to the extent that the blood supply to the foot may be compromised (anterior compartment syndrome).

More severe cases apparently result from irritation of the periosteum of the bone at the areas of origin of the front calf muscles and x-rays in these cases may, in time, show evidence of a periosteal reaction.

Treatment includes interdiction of the precipitating activity and the use of analgesics. The disability may be prolonged, especially for return to athletic activity. If pain is severe, even at rest, and there is acute tenderness over the anterior compartment, careful check must be made for evidence of diminished arterial supply to the foot. If there is any indication of vascular insufficiency, prompt referral should be made for possible surgical decompression of the anterior compartment.

CHAPTER 10
THE HIP (*)

Although hip conditions are not statistically represented in this compilation of compensable orthopaedic cases, the area does contain some features of interest to the occupational physician and nurse. Fractures about the hip are generally major and out of the scope of dispensary practice, but a knowledge of their clinical characteristics may be important in estimating the duration of disability and overall prognosis. The hip is a common site for degenerative arthritis which frequently requires permanent job restrictions or transfer to other work. Early recognition of the precursors may allow appropriate job placement in advance of the onset of symptoms so as to prevent or minimize disability.

Just as the shoulder symbolizes the dedication of the upper extremity to mobility, the hip epitomizes the stability which keynotes the function of the lower extremity. It is a true ball and socket joint. The deep, cup-shaped acetabulum is deepened still further by a fibro-cartilaginous rim so that the hip joint socket encloses more than three-quarters of the ball shaped head of the femur. The large area of contact between the two articular surfaces plus the pressures of weight bearing require perfect congruity between femoral head and acetabulum if the hip is to function painlessly through a working lifetime. A number of developmental abnormalities in the region of the hip adversely affect the congruity of the opposing joint surfaces. They are detectable at an age when most individuals are first entering the work force. They foretell future hip problems and should be seriously considered in determining the occupational future of the applicant.

FRACTURES (*)

All major fractures about the hip require expert hospital care. In the displaced fractures of the neck or intertrochanteric region of the femur, there is obvious shortening and helpless eversion of the affected leg and little problem with diagnosis. Splinting with a Thomas splint or with the legs strapped together and arrangements for transfer to the hospital are

119

all that is required.

Both fractures of the neck of the femur and those through the intertrochanteric area, however, may be undisplaced and the classical signs of broken hip may be absent. Even a routine x-ray of the injured hip may not be diagnostic. Usually, though, a 14 by 17 inch antero posterior view of the pelvis and both hips will allow the diagnosis to be made by comparing the injured with the uninjured hip. Care must be taken in positioning the patient for the x-ray that the legs are held in identical degrees of rotation. Figure 39 illustrates the value of this examination in the diagnosis of a fracture of the neck of the left femur and Figure 40 clearly shows an intertrochanteric fracture on the left. Both fractures might have been missed were the opposite hip not available for comparison. A missed early diagnosis in both cases might well have compromised the ultimate outcome.

Femoral Neck (*)

Fractures of the neck of the femur traverse bone with a poor blood

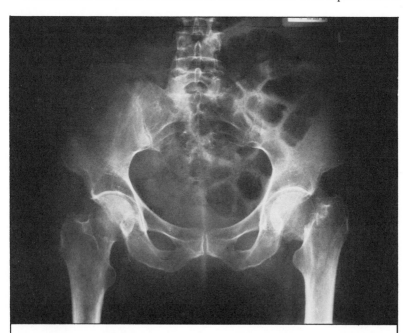

Figure 39. Anterio-posterior view of pelvis and both hips. Alteration in contour of neck of left femur (viewer's right) aids in the diagnosis of fracture of the femoral neck.

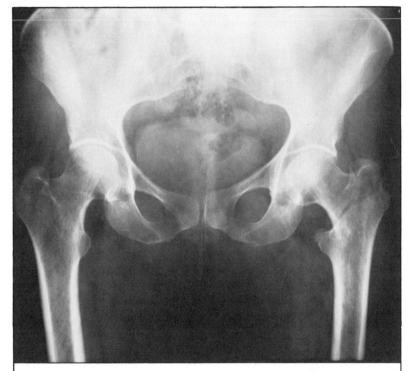

Figure 40. X-ray including pelvis and both hips allows easy identification of intertrochanteric fracture of the left femur (viewer's right).

supply and carry a guarded prognosis for uncomplicated bony union. Healing time is long (six to 12 months). Aseptic necrosis of the head and/or non-union may force secondary procedures. The likelihood of a return to work involving vigorous activity and extended periods of standing or walking is relatively slight.

Intertrochanteric (*)

Fractures in the intertrochanteric region involve bone with a much better blood supply than do femoral neck fractures. They are usually treated by internal fixation and the prognosis for bony union in three to six months is fairly good. The chances of a return to productive work are favorable although the patient may need to be protected from physically demanding jobs.

The prognosis depends upon the degree of damage to the acetabulum and the extent to which restoration is possible by traction or open reduction and internal fixation, and upon the fate of the blood supply to the head of the femur. In general, prognosis must be guarded and prosthetic replacement of one or both elements of the joint may have to be undertaken.

Acetabulum (*)

Most acetabular fractures are fracture-dislocations of the hip in which the femoral head is driven out the back of the acetabulum, breaking the posterior lip of the socket. Many result from motor vehicle accidents in which the knee is impacted against the dash-board and the thrust is delivered up the shaft of the femur to the hip.

DEVELOPMENTAL ABNORMALITIES (*)

Three types of developmental abnormalities affect the congruity of the hip joint and presage early degenerative arthritis.

1. **Acetabular dysplasia**
   May vary in degree from a small, shallow acetabulum to complete congenital dislocation of the hip, sometimes with the formation of a false acetabulum at some point higher up on the pelvis. May be bilateral. History of treatment in severe cases.

2. **Osteochondritis (Legg-Calve-Perthes disease)**
   Produces a flat, enlarged femoral head. Degenerative changes in the hip, symptomatic, are often present by the late teens or early twenties. Usually, history of treatment.

3. **Slipped upper femoral capital epihpysis**
   Produces a tear-drop shaped femoral head, posteriorly angulated. May be bilateral. In mild cases, may be no history of treatment and patient may not be aware of condition.

CHAPTER 11
THE PELVIS (1)

The two halves of the pelvis meet at the symphysis pubis in the midline anteriorly and join the keystone-shaped sacrum in the back to complete the pelvic ring. Upon the top of the sacrum rests the spine and all of the weight of the trunk, the head and the upper extremities. Apart from the occasional fracture, the chief orthopaedic interest in the pelvis lies in the manner in which it transmits forces to the low back. A lateral tilt of the pelvis, such as might result from difference in leg length, forces an angled take-off of the spine from the top of the sacrum and necessitates compensatory adjustments in order to center the head and upper trunk over the midline of the body. Similarly, a forward tilt of the pelvis, such as might occur in pregnancy or pot-belly obesity, imposes a forward-angled take-off of the spine from the top of the sacrum and this must be compensated for in the spine if the head is to end up reasonably well balanced over the center of gravity. In this situation, lumbar hyper-lordosis is the usual compensatory mechanism and may be a potent factor in low back pain.

The major bones of the pelvic ring are heavily ensheathed in the powerful muscles which take origin from it and are injured only in massive trauma, usually by body crush. Displaced fractures of the pelvic ring are life or death emergencies since there is likely to be associated damage to internal organs or major blood vessels. Major pelvis fractures have been reported second only to head injuries among the most common causes of traumatic death.

The lower portion of the sacrum, the coccyx and the iliac crests are more exposed and are subject to injury by less devastating impact. Because of the large number of muscles attached to the pelvis, avulsion fractures inevitably occur.

FRACTURES (1)

Avulsions (*)
Avulsion fractures of the pelvis are seen most commonly in youth and

123

usually in association with athletics. The ischial tuberosity may be pulled off by the hamstrings. The anterior inferior spine of the ileum is occasionally avulsed by one of the quadriceps insertions, usually in the act of kicking when the forward motion of the foot is suddenly impeded.

Treatment in avulsion fractures is largely symptomatic and the fracture fragments often unite by fibrous tissue, rather than bone.

Coccyx and Sacrum (*)
Fractures of the coccyx usually result from a sit-down fall, and are fairly common. Less frequently, the lower segments of the sacrum may be fractured in the same kind of accident. Both types of fractures are treated symptomatically. Because of irritation of the sacro-coccygeal plexus of nerves, these fractures may initiate long periods of symptomatic complaints.

Pelvic Ring (1)
Most common of the fractures involving the pelvic ring are those of one or both rami of the pubic bone anteriorly. These may be unilateral or bilateral, but usually are not significantly displaced. They may result from a relatively low impact front-to-back crush or even from a fall. They are seen more frequently in older patients who may have some degree of osteoporosis.

Although treatment is symptomatic, the initial degree of disability may be such as to require bed rest for a week or so. Ambulation with support may be started as soon as tolerated and bony healing is usually complete within six to eight weeks.

Displaced fractures of the pelvic ring must be assumed to have involved internal organs or major blood vessels until proved to the contrary. They usually result from heavy impact crush injuries. Blood pressure and pulse recordings should be started at once and repeated every 15 minutes while maintaining close observation for signs of shock. Massive blood loss can occur quickly and the hemorrhage be clinically hidden in the pelvis. There may also be injury to the bladder or urethra. If possible, a urine specimen should be obtained and examined for blood. Most importantly, however, the patient should be transported to the hospital as an emergency.

CHAPTER 12
THE NECK (10)

Slender, lightly muscled and highly mobile, the neck must support the considerable weight of the head, position it for best use of its sensory organs, and, at the same time, present a stable tube for the passage of the spinal cord. The conflicting demands for mobility and stability spell high vulnerability. Neck injuries must be regarded as potentially dangerous and handled with extreme caution.

There is a striking similarity in mechanics between the cervical and the lumbar segments of the spine, and the neck shares the characteristics of its typical attritional changes with the low back. Viewed from the side, the cervical spine is curved forward just as is the lumbar spine. The lower cervical vertebrae are the first mobile parts above a relatively fixed and immobile section of the spine, the thoracic region, just as the lower lumbar vertebrae are the first mobile segments above the fixed sacrum and pelvis. Degenerative changes occur early and often in the lower two cervical discs, just as they do in the lower two lumbar discs, and constitute the cause of a high percentage of neck pain. Just as low back pain is often accompanied by radicular phenomena in the legs, so are cervical complaints often associated with radiating pain, paraesthesias and weakness in the arms and hands.

SPRAINS AND STRAINS (6)

Injury usually occurs on sudden flexion of the neck, although this may be a recoil from a hyper-extension thrust. The weight of the head contributes momentum and there is stretching and tearing of ligaments in and around the facet joints combined with stretching and tearing of the relatively weak supporting cervical musculature. The typical injury is thus a blend of ligamentous sprain and muscular strain. The popular term, "whiplash neck", is descriptive and not entirely inappropriate.

As in other sprains, the key determination is the presence or absence of instability. Abnormal motion between the cervical vertebrae is detected by making lateral x-rays of the cervical spine in flexion and in extension. Such an examination is not without danger and it should be

125

made only after careful clinical evaluation of the extent of injury including a complete neurological appraisal. When in doubt, a single lateral x-ray of the cervical spine, which can be made in the supine position without moving the patient, may be helpful. If the normal anterior cervical curve is preserved, the chances of dangerous degrees of instability are relatively small. If the cervical spine is straight, indicating protective muscle spasm, the chance of significant damage is greater and strong consideration should be given to referral for expert opinion.

Treatment is determined by the degree of instability and may vary from a simple padded collar for a few days to hospitalization for traction followed by immobilization in a head-body cast or brace. Recovery, even in seemingly mild cases without evidence of instability, may be slow especially in cases involving litigation. Whip-lash necks resulting from low speed rear-end collisions have acquired the unsavory reputation of being cured only by green-back plasters.

FRACTURE DISLOCATION (1)

Fractures in the cervical spine are often accompanied by some degree of subluxation or dislocation of a vertebra. They frequently result from a fall, landing on the head, often in diving accidents. The external evidence of violence to the face and head can often be used as an indication of the probable degree of neck damage. Patients must be moved and handled with extreme care, the neck and head always supported and immobilized. Most ambulances now carry special immobilizing devices for neck injuries, but, until such a device can be applied, the neck must be stabilized manually.

Patients with any degree of neck pain following a fall on the head should be evaluated only in the hospital by experts.

AGGRAVATION OF PRE-EXISTING
DEGENERATIVE CHANGES (3)

Minor injuries may provoke severe neck and radicular symptoms in patients with pre-existing degenerative changes, which usually involve the lower cervical discs. As the result of disc degeneration there may be secondary facet joint degeneration with bony productive changes, narrowing of the neural foramina, and even instability between adjoining vertebrae exactly as occurs in the lower lumbar area.

Irritation of or pressure upon cervical nerve roots emerging from the spine at the levels of disc degeneration may produce confusing symptoms in the upper extremity. Pain in the shoulder area similar to that of rotator cuff tendinitis can be a radicular phenomenon. The symptoms of lateral epicondylitis, cross-over tendinitis and carpal tunnel syndrome, among others, can be mimicked by nerve root irritation secondary to pathological changes in the neck.

Usually, such radicular symptoms can be reproduced and aggravated by hyper-extension of the neck and by lateral flexion of the cervical spine toward the painful side with the application of sudden downward pressure on the head. In addition, in radicular symptomatology, the points of maximum tenderness are usually not precisely in the spots usually found in cases with primary local abnormality. Unilateral depression of the triceps, biceps or radio-periosteal reflexes or measurable atrophy of one arm may be found in cervical radiculopathy and assist in the differential diagnosis.

Treatment usually begins with physiotherapy including cervical traction and the use of a neck support. If supervised traction produces relief, the patient can be supplied with a head halter traction rig for use several times a day at home. Commercial collars for neck support are now made of plastic, velcro-fastened, and easily adjustable for individual fit. Their use should be strictly supervised since it is easy for patients to become dependent upon them and progressively lose supportive cervical musculature.

If symptoms are not controlled by conservative treatment, and if objective signs of nerve root pressure appear or increase, the patient should be referred for expert evaluation. Cervical myeolgraphy or electromyography may determine a need for cervical disc surgery. If there are indications for surgical treatment, intervertebral body fusion is often done.

Patients with symptomatic cervical disc degeneration often have trouble with jobs requiring constant or repetitive hyper-extension of the neck and may require job modification or transfer to other work.

CHAPTER 13
THE THORAX (25)

Comprised of the rib cage, the sternum and the thoracic and upper lumbar segments of the spine, the thoracic region is relatively immobile except for the pumping action of respiration. Expansion of the chest cavity for inspiration is produced by upward motion of the ribs at hinge joints with the vertebrae and by descent of the diaphragm. A form of arthritis of the spine (ankylosing spondylitis) often affects these costo-vertebral joints early in its course, and diminished chest expansion may be one of the first diagnostic signs of the disease.

The clinically important muscles of the area, apart from those associated with respiration, are mainly concerned with motion of the scapula on the rib cage as an adjunct to shoulder and arm function. These can be involved in acute strains but more frequently give rise to chronic symptoms in poorly designed work situations, postural problems or tension.

The thorax is most commonly injured by direct impact and most of the reported cases involve rib fractures or chest wall contusions. Fractures of vertebrae in the lower thoracic and upper lumbar regions of the spine, which are less common, occur by transmitted force in sudden forward jack-knifing of the body. The body of the vertebra is compressed into a wedge shape.

FRACTURES (12)

Ribs (10)
Rib fractures, often multiple, may occur at the point of impact in direct blows to the rib cage or at the area of maximum curve along the axillary line in crushing injuries of the chest. In either case, the trauma is likely to be significant and obvious. In the rare cases in which ribs are fractured by coughing, sneezing or sudden motion, there are usually pre-existing pathological changes in the bones, either severe osteoporosis or some type of primary or metastatic tumor.

129

On examination, there is generally severe local tenderness, well localized to one or more ribs, with pain on deep breathing which becomes excruciating upon coughing or sneezing. Compression of the rib cage by manual pressure exerted at two points well away from the area of tenderness will produce pain in the tender area.

The diagnosis of rib fracture is a clinical one since x-rays made soon after injury may not show a fracture line. Later x-rays may show callus and confirm, radiologically, the clinical diagnosis. The chief value of early x-rays is to exclude evidence of internal injury, usually represented by hemothorax or pneumothorax. The presence of such evidence automatically indicates hospitalization for observation and expert care.

In the uncomplicated case of rib fracture, external support to the rib cage is supplied in the form of adhesive strapping, elastic bandage wrap, or commercial rib belt. All produce reasonable comfort for the two to three week healing period. Since chest expansion will be limited for the duration of fracture healing, patients with chronic bronchial or lung disease must be observed carefully during the period of treatment.

Vertebra (2)

Fractures of vertebrae usually occur at the dorso-lumbar junction at or just above waist level and involve either the 11th or 12th thoracic or the first or second lumbar vertebrae (Figure 41). They result most commonly from injury which produces sudden forward flexion of the body at the waist. A fall, landing on the feet or the buttocks, is a common mechanism in industry. Outside of work, taking a jump on a toboggan or a snowmobile is a frequent cause as the patient jack-knifes forward upon impact to the buttocks in landing.

Most fractures involve anterior compression of the body of the vertebra and leave the posterior arch intact. Such fractures producing no more than 50 percent collapse of the front of the vertebral body do not generally pose a threat of instability or spinal cord damage and can usually be treated by the non-specialist.

Occasionally, there is difficulty with diagnosis. The patient may report with pain exclusively or predominantly in the low back, even though the injury is several segments higher. There may be tenderness to palpation over the lumbo-sacral area and it is easy to be misled into the belief that a low back injury has occurred. It is mandatory, therefore, that all patients with a suggestive history of injury have x-rays that include the lower dorsal and upper lumbar regions, even though complaints be maximum in, or restricted to, the low back area.

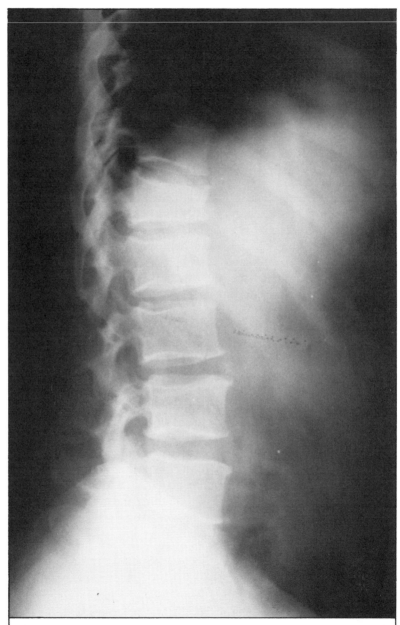

Figure 41. Typical compression fracture of the 12th thoracic vertebra. The body of the vertebra has been wedged anteriorly about 20 percent.

In injuries resulting from a fall, landing on the feet, it is well to examine the heels for evidence of calcaneal fracture and, conversely, in patients with calcaneal fracture, the possibility of compression fracture of the dorso-lumbar junction should be excluded by appropriate examination.

Providing the posterior arch of the vertebra is intact and the compression of the anterior portion of the vertebral body does not exceed 50 percent of its normal height, most of the compression fractures of the dorso-lumbar area are treated by early ambulation after an initial period of bed rest to relieve the acute symptoms. Retro-peritoneal bleeding of some degree usually accompanies these fractures and results in paralytic ileus with constipation, abdominal distension and discomfort. This generally clears within a few days and the patient can then be allowed to move about as tolerated. Instructions should be given in maintaining a straight and rigid spine, especially in shifting from the supine to the sitting and from the sitting to the standing position. External support in the form of a corset or brace may be necessary for a few weeks, although many patients with mild compressions do not require this. Healing time is from 16 to 20 weeks and, during this time, the patient should do no work requiring bending or lifting.

In mild compressions, there may be no significant permanency providing early ambulation has been possible and weakness and atrophy of the supportive musculature of the trunk has not occurred. Severe compressions may so increase the posterior convexity of the lower thoracic spine as to require increases in the lumbar and cervical lordoses in order to bring the head back on center over the pelvis. Chronic pain, usually in the low back, may result.

Fractures of the thoracic spine above the 10th thoracic vertebra are relatively rare because of the splinting action of the ribs. When they do occur, they usually result from massive trauma and are but one feature of a medley of serious injuries.

STRAINS (4)

Muscle strains in the region of the thorax usually involve the trapezius, the latissimus dorsi or the rhomboids. While occasionally seen after acute injury, they are more likely to present as chronic, low-grade muscle aches relating to postural problems or to tension. They are fairly common among typists and computer keyboard operators who may sit for long hours, bent over their machines with the arms suspended. Long-necked, slope-shoulded individuals are part-icularly prone to chronic strains of the trapezius and rhomboid muscles.

Treatment, in addition to analgesics, may involve alterations in work chairs or the chair-to-keyboard position, arrangments to allow frequent rest breaks and a regime of physiotherapy and corrective exercises. Trigger spots in the involved muscles develop fairly frequently and often respond well to local injection with novacaine. It is sometimes necessary to transfer patients with persistent complaints out of high pressure, deadline types of jobs in order to reduce the tension which often figures prominently in the symptom pattern.

CONTUSIONS (5)

Contusions of the chest wall result from the same mechanism of injury and have the same presenting complaints as rib fractures, but have no clinical or x-ray findings confirmatory of fracture. Treatment is symptomatic and may be the same as for rib fracture with the use of rib cage support for a week or ten days.

SPRAINS (3)

Sprains in the thorax region usually involve the joints between the ribs and the sternum (costo-sternal joints) or those between the bony and cartilaginous portions of the lower ribs (costo-chondral junction). Treatment is similar to that for rib fractures with the use of a rib belt or other external rib cage support. Symptoms may become chronic and are often associated with enlargement of the costo-chondral junction or the costo-sternal joint. In such cases, local injection with novacaine and steroids is frequently effective. Even when complete symptomatic relief is achieved, however, there is a fairly high incidence of recurrent symptoms on resumption of vigorous activity. Athletes, particularly those involved in heavy arm and shoulder sports, may experience recurrent symptoms from rib cage sprains over a period of many months.

CHAPTER 14
THE LOW BACK (257)

The Frequency Index of 257, while impressive, tells only part of the story of low back problems in industry. In addition to being common, they are inordinately expensive.

Nationwide, back cases constitute about 20 percent of all compensation cases, but account for more than 33 percent of total dollars spent for Workers' Compensation claims. The overage in costs is attributable to a relatively small number of cases which progress to long term disability. It is estimated that 15 percent of low back patients account for 80 percent of the costs.

The great majority of patients with attacks of low back pain either lose no time from work or are back on the job within two or three weeks. Their average costs are about the same as for other conditions of the same duration.

Identification of the potential long term disability case and early effective intervention is of paramount importance if the low back problem in industry is to be controlled. Low back disability has well-established points of no return. There is only a 50 percent chance that a patient who has been off the job for six months with a back problem will ever return to work. Extend the disability period to 12 months and the chance of a return drops to 25 percent. Beyond two years of disability, the chances of ever returning to productive employment are practically nil.

In each of the anatomical areas described in foregoing chapters, it has been possible, by thoughtful consideration of the structural characteristics of the region and of the functional demands imposed upon it, to foretell the clinical conditions likely to occur, and, with the help of solid objective findings from examination and x-ray, to predict with fair accuracy the degree and duration of disability. Not so with the low back.

It is true that the architecture, mechanical stresses and attritional characteristics of the low back region forecast a high incidence of structural failure and backache, but there is only scanty and unreliable objective evidence upon which to base an estimate of disability. The same degree of low back abnormality, as nearly as can be defined by even the most sophisticated diagnostic tools and techniques, may translate to an annoyance in one patient, a disastrous disability in another. Only recently have serious studies been directed at the crucial question in low back troubles—the determination of disability.

Coping with low back problems requires not only an understanding of the pathomechanics of the area, but a clear perception of a wide variety of disability determinants, many of which have little or nothing to do with the condition of the low back, itself.

Nowhere is it so important to know the whole patient. Elements in individual make-up as simple as age, general medical condition, level of intelligence and training or as complex as motivation, innate resilience and general psychological sets may play major roles in disability determination.

In no other orthopaedic problem at work is an intimate knowledge of the environment in which the patient works and lives more essential. Considerations as obvious as the physical demands of the job, the work record and the benefit schedule or as abstruse as the level of job satisfaction, of relationships with supervisors and fellow workers, attitudes toward the employer and the situation at home may be the real determinants of wellness or illness.

STRUCTURE, FUNCTION AND PATHOMECHANICS

The fact that about 80 percent of people will, on one or more occasions during their lifetimes, have backache suggests that the architecture of the spine may not meet functional demands or that the basic building materials may lack durability for the average life span and usage of the assembly. Examination of the structure of the low back in relation to the known stresses to which it is subjected is helpful in explaining the frequent break-downs.

The spine is a vertical assembly of 24 separate bones, the vertebrae, mounted on a base, the pelvis and sacrum, which slopes forward about 40 degrees from the horizontal (Figure 42). Viewed from the side, there are three reciprocal curves which are necessary to bring the center of gravity of the upper body and head over the pelvic base. In the full upright position, the entire assembly is in a state of dynamic balance and little muscular effort is required to maintain equilibrium. Most human activities, however, require some forward inclination of the trunk, often with weight held in the hands at variable distances forward of the center of gravity. Once forward flexion of the trunk occurs, a

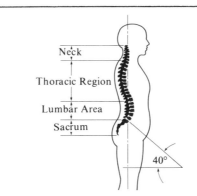

Neck

Thoracic Region

Lumbar Area

Sacrum

40°

Figure 42. The Human Spine. The base (sacrum bone of the pelvis) upon which the jointed assembly of vertebrae mount is sloped forward from the horizontal plane about 40°. The resulting angled take-off of the spine from the pelvis is compensated for by three reciprocal curves (convexity forward in the lumbar area, convexity backward in the thoracic region, and convexity forward in the neck). This brings the center of gravity of the head and upper body over the pelvic base in a state of dynamic equilibrium.

considerable amount of muscle work is required to maintain the desired position against the force of gravity and significant increases in pressure are created, mainly at the junction between the jointed rod of the spine and its fixed base, the pelvis and sacrum. Simply bending forward 45 degrees or so to brush one's teeth over the lavatory or leaning over a drafting board generates pressures at the lumbo-sacral junction upwards of 600 pounds. Bend forward 90 degrees and lift a 65 pound weight and the pressure soars to more than 1500 pounds. With pressures of this magnitude, rules of engineering design would dictate at least a horizontal shelf upon which to base the load. Such, however, is not the case in the human low back where the forward slope of the top of the sacrum translates to a significant degree of shearing stress in the region of the lumbo-sacral junction. It is in this area that most low back problems occur.

The 24 vertebrae comprising the spine are coupled, one to the next, in such a way as to allow a limited range of motion to occur between each two segments. This coupling is a three-point suspension system. The spool-like bodies of the vertebrae are jointed together by the inter-vertebral disc and the posterior arches by a pair of facet joints formed by the junction between the inferior articular processes of the vertebra above and the superior articular processes of the vertebra below (Figure 43).

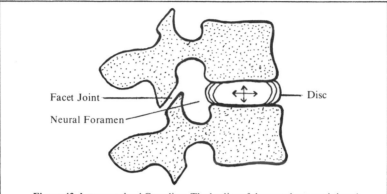

Facet Joint

Neural Foramen

Disc

Figure 43. Intervertebral Coupling. The bodies of the vertebrae are jointed together by the intervertebral disc and the posterior arches by paired facet joints (right and left) formed by the junction between the inferior articular processes of the vertebra above and the superior articular processes of the vertebra below. The rounded space between the two vertebrae is the neural foramen or port hole for exit of the nerve roots which branch from the spinal cord.

In the normal state, the major weight of the trunk is carried by the vertebral bodies and the interposed intervertebral discs. The facet joints bear only token weight and serve chiefly to determine the direction of motion, which varies from one region of the spine to another. Motion between each two vertebrae must be accomplished without any slipping or sliding of one vertebra upon the next because of the vulnerable position of the spinal cord, which runs down the bony tunnel created by the jointed posterior arches of the vertebrae, and of its branching nerve roots, which exit the spinal tunnel through right and left port holes between each two vertebrae (neural foramina).

The range of motion in the lumbar region of the spine is limited largely to flexion and extension, but is considerable in degree as shown in Figure 44. Although the vertebrae are bound together by a large number of ligaments, it is clear that, were the ligaments sufficiently snug to prevent fore-and-aft or side-to-side motion of one vertebra upon another, this range of motion could not occur. The important job of maintaining alignment and stability between vertebrae throughout this motion range is assigned to the intervertebral disc, and the ligaments serve only as check-reins against motion beyond the designed limits of the unit.

Long regarded as a simple shock absorber, the intervertebral disc emerges as the chief stabilizer of the spine and the guardian against

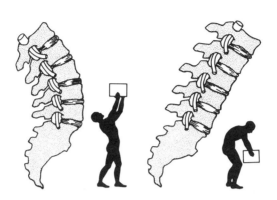

Figure 44. Range of motion in lumbar spine. The lumbar spine is capable of bending backward to a point where the spinous processes almost touch and forward sufficiently to reverse the normal lumbar lordosis. Note nerve roots exiting from the spinal canal through neural foramina between each two vertebrae.

abnormal motion between the vertebrae which could produce mechanical irritation or actual pinching of the spinal cord or its nerve root branches.

The intervertebral disc is made up of an outer casing of fibro-elastic tissue attached circumferentially to the margins of the bodies of adjoining vertebrae and an inner chamber packed with a gel-like substance under positive pressure. Somewhat simplistically, its stabilizing role can be visualized as the expanding force of the pressurized packing constantly pushing the adjoining vertebral bodies apart to the full extent allowed by the casing fibers in whatever position the spine may be operating. Much more than a shock absorber, the disc is a unique pressurized hydraulic flexible coupler, vital to the painless function of the spine.

Discs work well and are reasonably durable when loading is fairly uniform across their horizontal surfaces, as occurs in the upper lumbar and thoracic segments of the spine. When there is tilting away from the horizontal such as occurs in the lower lumbar region, however, elements of shearing stress which are poorly tolerated by such structures are introduced and, moreover, loading is concentrated upon one small arc of the total circumference in the posterior third of the disc. The disc fails most commonly posteriorly at the fourth and fifth lumbar levels.

Here, the hundreds of pounds of pressure generated by normal daily activities ultimately exact their toll in the form of microscopic stretchings, tearings and ravelings of the casing fibers. The casing of the disc is avascular and, like the rotator cuff tendons of the shoulder, incapable of repair. The increments of micro-damage become cumulative until, finally, the casing is no longer capable of containing the pressure of the packing material. Usually, slow leaks of the fluid content of the gel packing occur from time to time and the disc begins to narrow and gradually go flat. Less commonly, the weakened casing may bulge or a sudden blow-out may occur and a massive amount of the packing material may suddenly herniate through a large tear in the casing, exerting pressure against the nerve root in its bony port hole and creating the classical ruptured disc.

In the usual scenario of slow disc degeneration, the loss of competence of the prime stabilizer leads to a sequence of secondary effects which are responsible for a broad range of clinical manifestations (Figure 45). In the three-point suspension system, loss of height of the disc, the anterior suspension member, causes a corresponding loss of height at the two posterior suspension points, the facet joints. The articular processes of the adjoining vertebrae ride past one another (sublux). The inclination of the facet joints dictates that the upper vertebra drop backwards as well as downwards on the vertebra below. The subluxation of the facet joint narrows the horizontal diameter of the port hole as the upper tip of the superior articular process of the lower vertebra creates a bony bulge in the middle of the space, posteriorly (Figure 45B). Since the upper vertebral body has also settled backward as well as downward, the posterior inferior corner of the body of the vertebra also invades the nerve root port from the front. The vertical diameter of the port has already been decreased by the settling of the whole suspension system so the space for the nerve root is both constricted and distorted and the margin of safety for the nerve root is reduced to a critical point.

In addition, the stability between the two vertebrae has been lost with the loss of pressure in the disc packing, and slipping of one vertebra upon another with motion of the trunk can now occur. Sooner or later, mechanical irritation or episodes of actual pinching of the nerve root are all but inevitable (Figure 45C).

As the disc narrows and gradually goes flat, more and more weight falls upon the facet joints, which are not designed for weight bearing and which have already subluxed. Traumatic arthritic degeneration ensues and may result in its own set of distinctive symptoms.

Finally, the process of disc degeneration terminates as scar tissue,

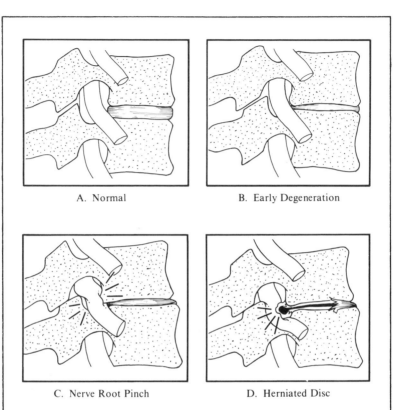

A. Normal   B. Early Degeneration

C. Nerve Root Pinch   D. Herniated Disc

Figure 45. The Pathomechanics of Disc Degeneration.
   (A) Normal state.
   (B) Early degeneration. The disc space has narrowed, forcing
       over-riding of the articular processes at the facet joint.
       Because of the inclination of the facet joints, the body of the
       top vertebra settles backward as well as downward on the
       body of the lower vertebra. The port of exit for the nerve
       root (neural foramen) loses vertical height and its horizontal
       configuration becomes distorted with reduction in the
       margin of safety for the nerve root. The disc has lost internal
       pressure, its casing fibers have become slack and there is
       potential slipping of one vertebra upon the other.
   (C) Further narrowing of the disc space, subluxation of the facet
       joint, constriction and distortion of the neural foramen and
       loss of stability between vertebrae may now allow occasional
       pinching of the nerve root with motion of the spine.
   (D) Herniated or ruptured disc. The casing has blown out
       allowing the remaining gel packing to extrude and impinge
       upon the nerve root.

which has been slowly building up in the packing chamber, becomes strong enough to lash the adjoining vertebrae together in a fibrous union. Motion at this segment gradually diminishes and symptoms gradually decline and may all but disappear as intervertebral stability is regained.

Disc rupture, which occurs in less than 10 percent of patients with degenerative disc disease, is most likely to occur during the thirties or forties when, presumably, the patient is old enough to have developed significant weakening of the casing, but young enough to have a relatively high fluid content in the gel packing (Figure 45D).

The whole process of disc degeneration may take more than thirty years from the first increments of micro-damage to the casing, which usually begin in the twenties, through the gradual narrowing and secondary mechanical adjustments of the thirties and forties, the degenerative facet joint changes which ordinarily produce symptoms in the early fifties, to the final scarring and relative comfort of the late fifties and sixties.

Disc degeneration in one of its several phases is now generally conceded to be the most common cause of low back troubles, accounting for nearly 70 percent of the cases seen in industry.

THE CLINICAL PICTURE

Symptoms vary with the age of the patient and the stage of the degenertive process. During the twenties, when damage to the casing fibers is most apt to begin, there are intermittent attacks of acute low back pain of relatively short duration. These attacks usually begin suddenly, sometimes in association with some unusual activity or sudden exertion, but, as often as not, simply in the course of normal activity. Seldom is there a history of impressive trauma. The pain may be sufficiently severe to require work restriction or even a few days off the job. Symptoms clear completely after a week or ten days and the patient returns to full normal activity without any residual.

After several months or even a few years of complete freedom from symtoms, there is likely to be another attack, much like the first but usually a little more severe and lasting a bit longer. Again, symptoms clear fairly promptly.

Recurrent attacks then occur with increasing frequency, severity and duration. By the late twenties or early thirties, the pain, instead of being diffuse across the entire low back, becomes lateralized to one side or the other and there may be radiation into the corresponding buttock.

Symptoms are slower to disappear and there may be some residual ache, off and on, between acute attacks. Succeeding attacks through the thirties and into the forties are accompanied by more and more radiation of pain, first into the back of the thigh, then into the calf and, finally, shooting all the way down the back of the leg into the foot. There may be numbness of the side of the calf or the foot and perhaps some weakness in raising the foot.

These attacks, featuring radicular pain in the leg, occur as the nerve root exiting the spinal canal at the level of disc failure suffers mechanical irritation or even momentary pressure because of the abnormal motion between the adjoining vertebrae. Unless there has been an actual rupture of the casing with protrusion of packing material impinging the nerve root, such attacks will clear with conservative treatment, but over a considerably longer period of time than in the attacks of the younger years. The nerve root, having been irritated or pinched, swells and may develop a secondary inflammatory reaction. A period of bed rest and, perhaps, anti-inflammatory medication is necessary to allow the swollen and engorged nerve root to shrink back to normal size.

The decades of the thirties and forties are the most threatening times for disc disease and disability is most likely to occur during these years. In one industrial study, men in their thirties and forties who constituted 46 percent of the work force accounted for 71 percent of all lost time from work attributable to low back conditions.

As the patient enters the late forties and early fifties, the symptom pattern often changes. Acute attacks diminish in frequency and severity, but chronic arthritic symptoms apear and the patient may have low-grade backache much of the time. There may be stiffness of the back, especially upon arising in the morning, pain in cold, damp weather and poor tolerance to heavy physical activity. The backache of this age period is attributable to the degenerative arthritic changes in the subluxed and over-stressed facet joints.

Finally, in the late fifties and sixties, back trouble of significant degree diminishes and may disappear entirely. This period coincides with the re-establishment of stability of the intervetebral segment by scar tissue bridging the old packing chamber of the disc.

It should be noted that this clinical picture is but a sketchy outline of the scenario of degenerative disc disease. It advances from Act I, the time of the accumulation of micro-damage to the casing, through Act II, the period of nerve root involvement, into Act III, when facet joint arthritis makes its appearance, and, finally, into Act IV, the happy ending of scar re-stabilization of the intervertebral segment. Not all actors are on stage for the entire drama. Some appear in Act I and are never seen again. Some do not make their entrance until Act II, the most exciting and challenging period of the play. A few are only seen in Act III. Furthermore, all actors do not follow the script exactly and may play their roles slightly out of sync with the scenario. Attacks indicative of early casing damage may occur in the teens. Disc ruptures are not unknown in the fifties, or even the sixties. Some actors add highly individual interpretations of their roles and may stray away from the script, causing a certain amount of confusion for the stage manager. There is evidence that some individuals play out the whole drama of disc degeneration in symptomatic silence or, at least with so little reaction that they stay in the wings and never appear on stage at all. Taken as an outline of the action and not as a detailed script, however, the typical clinical picture is a distinct aid in following the complicated story.

DIAGNOSIS

Accurate determination of the cause or causes of low back pain in the individual patient is extremely difficult and, for the majority of younger patients in the early phases of degenerative disc disease, may be impossible to establish on the basis of objective findings. A glance at the outline of possible causes of low back pain in Table 4 gives some indication of the difficulty. The problem is further complicated by the frequent presence of multiple causes for backache in the same patient. Low back pain is often a brew of many ingredients and complete diagnosis may require the composition of a whole recipe rather than the detection of a single cause.

A bony structural abnormality such as spondylolisthesis, for instance, may never cause pain until the patient becomes pregnant or develops pot-belly obesity and thereby sumperimposes a functional abnormality upon the existing structural defect. Even the two causes may give no problems until a third cause such as loss of trunk muscle strength resulting from a period of physical inactivity enters the picture and finally precipitates symptoms.

Objective findings from physical examination, x-rays or laboratory tests are often sparse, frequently non-specific and seldom diagnostic. Even the true severity of the condition is difficult to quantify because of the wide variation in individual patient response to seemingly similar degrees of pathological changes in the low back. This variance in

POSSIBLE CAUSES OF LOW BACK PAIN

A. Referred Pain From Abdominal or Pelvic Organs
 1. Urinary Tract (kidney, ureter, bladder, prostate)
 2. Gastro-Intestinal Tract (ileum, colon, rectum)
 3. Female Genital System (uterus, ovaries, cervix)
 4. Vascular System (aneurism, arterial insufficiency)

B. Pain Originating in the Spine
 1. Abnormalities of Bony Structure
    a. Segmentation errors (4 or 6 lumbar, transitional vertebrae)
    b. Ossification defects (spondylolysis, spondylolisthesis)
    c. Dimension and angulation defects
 2. Functional abnormality
    a. Antero-posterior trunk imbalance (pregnancy, pot-belly obesity, pelvic tilt, poor workplace design)
    b. Lateral trunk imbalance (spine curvature, hearing or vision impairment, poor workplace design)
    c. Loss of strength in supportive musculature
 3. Inflammation
    a. Systemic infection or toxicity
    b. Infection of bones or joints (osteomyelitis, tuberculosis)
    c. Arthritis (ankylosing spondylitis, rheumatoid)
 4. Metabolic or hormonal
    a. Osteoporosis (post-menopausal, hyperthyroid or parathyroid)
    b. Diabetes, gout, Paget's disease
 5. Degenerative (discs, facet joints)
 6. Tumor
    a. Primary of bone (multiple myeloma, hemangioma, etc.)
    b. Primary of spinal cord or nerve roots
    c. Metastatic from other organs (breast, lung, prostate, etc.
 7. Injury
    a. Fracture of vertebral bodies or processes
    b. Sprains (ligaments) and strains (muscles)
    c. Acute rupture of disc

Table 4. Possible Causes of Low Back Pain

response may reflect the psychological make-up of the patient or may stem from elements in the complex socio-economic environment in which most industrial low back pain is seen.

Acute Low Back Pain

The occupational physician or nurse in day-to-day dispensary practice will be confronted more frequently with acute episodes of low back pain than with the chronic condition. The typical patient with acute low back pain is relatively young and usually presents with a history of sudden onset of severe, grabbing pain across the low back which has appeared without warning during the course of normal activity. Often the pain appears on straightening up after a period of working in a crouched position. A combination of lifting and twisting the trunk, as in swinging luggage into the trunk of a car, is a fairly common trigger. Sudden, unexpected moves, as in turning quickly to catch a falling object or having a carried load shift or slip may initiate the pain. Even a cough or a sneeze may precipitate an attack. Most often, though, the honest patient is unable to relate the onset of symptoms to any specific mechanical event.

A one year analysis of all low back patients reporting to the company dispensary showed that 68 percent were unable to ascribe their low back pain to any specific cause. Only 32 percent attributed symptoms to a specific incident. Half of these cited injury at work.

If there is a history of injury, it is important to understand the full details of the incident in order to make judgement as to the degree of tissue damage sustained. This requires knowledge of the weight of the load, its position relative to the body, where it was being lifted or lowered from and to, the time between the incident and the appearance of symptoms, the time of day (before warm-up or after onset of fatigue), the day of the week (high incidence of back complaints on Mondays), and the relationship, if any, to periods of time away from this particular activity (vacation, sick period, job rotation, etc.) and consequent loss of conditioning.

The medical record should be searched and the patient questioned concerning previous similar attacks. A history of such attacks in the past, especially with complete recovery between attacks, suggests early degenerative disc disease.

Physical examination is seldom of much assistance in diagnosing acute low back pain. The findings are likely to reflect the level of pain and incapacity rather than the cause of the difficulty. All back motions will be restricted and painful and straight leg raising will be limited by pain. The patient may be tilted to one side or the trunk held in a rigidly flexed position due to muscle spasm.

If there is radiation of pain into the leg, a careful neurological examination should be carried out for evidence of nerve root pressure. In an early disc attack, such signs are likely to be subtle. Depression of the ankle reflex on the painful side may not be detected if the patient is examined in the usual manner, sitting on the examining table with the legs dangling over the side. In this position, the lumbar spine is flexed and the nerve root ports are opened to their maximum. Performing the examination with the patient kneeling in a chair and bringing the back into a position of maximum hyperextension may yield a positive finding since, in this position, the neural foramina are squeezed tight and may exert pressure on the nerve root.

There is unlikely, at this stage, to be measurable atrophy of the calf or thigh or visable shrinking of the buttock musculature, but these should be checked. Slight weakness of dorsi-flexion of the great toe on the affected side as compared with the normal is occasionally a useful early sign of nerve root involvement.

Patients with any evidence of nerve root involvement must be treated carefully and observed closely for evidence of progression or regression of the neurological signs. Referral for specialist care may be indicated.

X-ray examination is not likely to be of much help in acute low back pain unless the history indicates the possibility of fracture, in which case it is important to include views of the dorso-lumbar junction as well as of the low back. In most cases, x-rays are deferred at least until muscle spasm has cleared, since the presence of muscle spasm makes it difficult to obtain films of good diagnostic quality. Unless there is a definite history of significant injury, delayed recovery or some unusual clinical feature, x-rays are often not taken at all in acute low backache.

Certain laboratory tests may be indicated in the acute low back patient depending upon the history. Urinary symptoms accompanying or preceding the back pain may dictate urinalysis to aid in the detection of urinary tract infection. Palpation of the prostate may be similarly indicated in such cases. If there is a suggestion that the backache may be related to systemic infection, the white blood cell and differential count and the sedimentation rate may be helpful.

Most acute low back pain is treated on the basis of history and an abbreviated examination and is carried through without the use of other diagnostic tools and, usually, without a definite diagnosis.

   Inability to establish a solid diagnosis underlies many of the problems
in the management of low back disability in industry. In order to meet
the legal requirement of Workers' Compensation laws, some diagnosis
must usually be recorded within hours of the onset of symptoms for the
patient whose backache has begun at work and is therefore deemed
compensable on the basis of having arisen "out of and in the course of
employment." Lacking specific findings, as is so often the case in acute
low back pain, diagnoses of low back sprain or strain are likely to be
made, even though no injury capable of stretching or tearing ligament
or muscle fibers can be identified. Such diagnoses of expediency, quite
apart from being inaccurate, may initiate a number of undesirable
reactions and create statistical misinformation with regard to the true
nature of the low back problem.
   An immediate credibility gap is created with regard to the veracity of
the patient and the validity of complaints if a diagnosis implying injury
is reported when supervisors and fellow-workers are reasonably sure
that no injury has occurred. Patients may have to shoulder overt or
covert expressions of doubt and suspicion on top of backache.
Perceiving themselves blameless in this legalistic charade, many
patients will react with anger toward the company and its representatives
and some will exaggerate or prolong disability in order to salvage self
respect or punish the system.
   On a larger scale, reported diagnoses implying injury have hampered
the effort to control low back disability in the working population,
fostering the notion that most backache in the workplace is traumatic in
origin and therefore can be prevented by approaches which are
applicable to other industrial injuries. For more than 50 years, serious
attempts have been made by Industry to prevent backache in the
workplace. These have included pre-placement screenings, sometimes
with x-rays of the low back, in an attempt to identify those susceptible
to back injury, extensive training of employees in safe methods of
lifting, provision of mechanical lifting aids, control of the weight of
loads to be lifted and safety campaigns agains back injuries.
   Despite the expenditure of thousands of dollars and countless hours
of thought and effort, worldwide statistics show no decrease in the
incidence or severity of low back problems. As an occasional side effect
of the dismal failure of these approaches and the frustration associated
with it, the patient who develops back pain at work shortly after having
been trained in safe lifting or in the midst of a safety campaign may well
be blamed for his backache on the basis of non-compliance or failure to

cooperate. Even the most loyal employee, suffering the frightening pain of acute low backache, sensing doubt as to the validity of his complaints, and then being blamed for developing them may well elect retributory moves against the employer.

If there are no findings from history or examination allowing a definite diagnosis to be made it is probably best to record, simply "low back pain" as the diagnosis. If the history and findings are those of an early disc attack, as will often be the case, it is proper to enter as a diagnosis "aggravation of a pre-existing condition - degenerative disc disease."

Legislators and legal experts are becoming increasingly aware of the ambiguities of low back pain in the workplace, attempting to decide whether it should be handled under the rubric of injury, as at present, or illness and, if illness, whether as occupational or non-occupational in nature. Clarification of the situation will ultimately occur, but, for the present, every attempt must be made to operate within current laws without doing gross injustice to the patient or thwarting attempts to understand and control this most vexing and expensive of Industry's medical problems.

Chronic Low Back Pain

In patients with chronic or recurrent low back pain, there is a much greater possibility of making a definite diagnosis. The average patient is older and has usually had backache over a sufficiently long period of time to have established a symptom pattern, which is helpful in suggesting probable diagnosis. Examination findings are more likely to be specific for disease rather than, as in acute attacks, representing simply reaction to pain. The x-ray examination may be of real value when correlated with the symptom patterns and the physical findings. Laboratory tests can supply critical diagnostic data in this group of patients.

Using the information in Table 4 as a check-list, a primary and, perhaps, one or more secondary diagnoses can usually be made. Fairly often, the pathological process underlying the primary diagnosis is not curable but the correction of secondary contributory abnormalities may so reduce the overall symptom level as to allow nearly normal function with significant reduction in discomfort.

In addition to identifying the primary cause of the back problem and recognizing the significant contributing abnormalities, the most useful diagnostic statement will estimate the probable impact of the low back pain upon the individual patient, taking into consideration such elements as age, level of general physical fitness, vocational assets, inherent physical and psychic make-up and motivation, and the interplay of factors in the work and home environment.

TREATMENT

Distinction is made between the medical treatment of low back pain and the management of low back disability in industry. The medical treatment of backache is relatively simple and straightforward. The intelligent mangement of low back disability is extremely complex and is a function, not just of medical people, but of all those in the industrial establishment who interface with the patient. It is the subject of a separate section.

Acute Low Back Pain

The first and most important objective in the treatment of acute low back pain is to relieve pain and anxiety. Especially in the first severe attack, the patient is frightened by the sudden and severe seizing pain of muscle spasm which strikes with any attempt to move. There is great need for reassurance as to the short duration of the acute phase of such attacks, and for ample doses of pain medication.

The patient is often first seen in the throes of the pain-spasm cycle, a reflex protective mechanism which, once triggered in the low back, is capable of self-perpetuation for periods of up to three or four days. The pain-spasm reflex is the mechanism which produces the board-like abdomen of acute appendicitis and which immobilizes serious extremity injuries within a few minutes. The muscles in the region of damage or disease involuntarily contract with maximum strength to freeze and immobilize the area, presumably to protect it against further damage.

In the low back, the protective muscles are thick and maximal prolonged contraction in spasm may, of itself, cause pain because the heavy muscles, in effect, clamp off their own blood supply. The result is somewhat like the pain of muscle cramp in the heavy calf muscles. The muscle pain evokes more spasm, the spasm begets more pain, and so, on and on, until the muscles become so fatigued that they no longer respond to motor impulses from the reflex center. The pain-spasm cycle may persist as the proximate cause of incapacity long after the triggering event has ceased to cause pain.

The pain-spasm cycle must be broken as quickly as possible and this is best accomplished by bed rest and the use of adequate analgesia. The patient who demonstrates muscle spasm of such degree that there is list of the trunk or inability to stand straight should be on absolute bed rest for 48 to 72 hours with regular use of pain medication. The most comfortable position in bed is likely to be the low Fowler's position, acheived by raising the upper part of the mattress about 30 degrees and placing a bolster of some sort under the knees. During sleep, the patient automatically assumes this position, lying on the side with the back, hips and knees slightly flexed in a semi-foetal position. The commercial lounger chair can produce a similar position. Some patients elect to sleep lying on the floor with the hips and knees flexed 90 degrees, the lower legs resting on a bed or chair.

Physiotherapy has little place in the treatment of the acute phase. Local heat application makes about half of patients worse, possibly by increasing the metabolic demands of muscles already operating with an insufficient blood supply. Ice massage has been advocated, and it may produce a local anaesthetic effect with temporary relief, but the effect is brief and it does not seem to shorten the total duration of the pain-spasm cycle.

After spasm has ceased, the back muscles will be tender and sore, but no longer hyper-irritable and subject to the sudden painful spasms. In this phase of recovery, local heat may be comforting, but can be conveniently applied at home by the use of hot tub baths or a heating pad. In general, in acute low back pain, formal physiotherapy is not worth the moving about necessary to get to and from the facility.

As muscle spasm subsides, a knee-to-chest exercise (Figure 46A) may be started in bed. At first with assistance, the hips and knees are slowly flexed until the thighs approximate the chest. Most patients find this maneuver comfortable and, if so, they may perform it actively as a regular exercise four or five times each waking hour. It has the double benefit of stretching the lumbar spine in flexion, tending to open the neural foramina posteriorly, and providing active exercise of the abdominal muscles, which are important stabilizers of the spine. The patient should be cautioned to skid the feet along the bed until the knees and hips are well flexed before lifting the legs onto the body and to return to the starting position by dropping the feet to the bed first and straightening the legs by sliding the feet along the bed surface. Lifting or lowering the straight legs will almost certainly be painful at this stage and may delay recovery from the acute attack. Some patients, who have experienced several acute attacks, find that an attack can be aborted or its severity significantly decreased by immediately performing the knee-

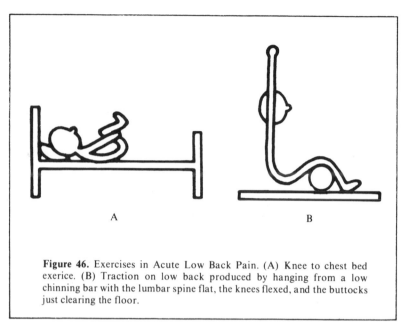

A   B

Figure 46. Exercises in Acute Low Back Pain. (A) Knee to chest bed
exerice. (B) Traction on low back produced by hanging from a low
chinning bar with the lumbar spine flat, the knees flexed, and the buttocks
just clearing the floor.

to-chest press with the first warning jabs of pain.

Many patients obtain relief during the early recovery phase by the
self-applied home use of body traction (Figure 46B). They hang by their
hands from a low chinning bar, temporarily installed in a door-way, in a
sitting position so that the buttocks just clear the floor. The knees rest
on bolsters or pillows allowing the patient to assume the position of
flexion of trunk, hips and knees which is most comfortable in bed. The
weight of the buttocks and thighs provides the traction. The patient
hangs for a few moments four or five times a day with relief that often
persists for several hours after each traction session.

For such moving about out of bed as is absolutely necessary, the
patient is advised to use crutches, since this takes the weight of the upper
body off the low back. Lacking crutches, the back of a straight chair can
be used for upper body support, the patient pushing the chair along in
front of him for more comfortable ambulation.

As the patient recovers from the acute attack, a simple exercise
program aimed at strengthening the abdominal muscles and stretching
the hamstrings is introduced (Figure 47). Recovery from the typical
acute attack is usually so swift and so complete, however, that the
average patient pays little attention to advice regarding special exercises.
Neither is the recovered acute low back patient, as a rule, receptive to

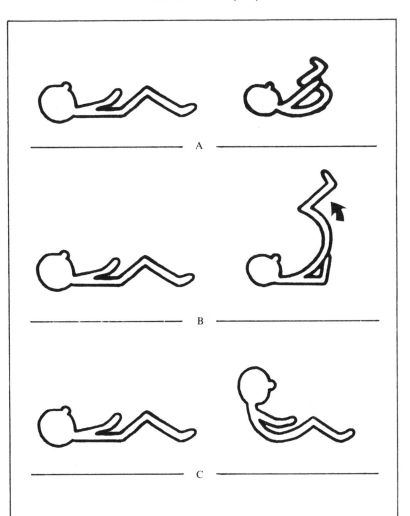

Figure 47. Exercises in Chronic Low Back Pain. (A) Knee to chest press. From start position, hips and knees are flexed, feet together, and knees squeezed tight against the chest. Lumbar spine is stretched in flexion. Abdominal muscles are used to raise the flexed legs onto the body. (B) Roll-Up Hamstring Stretch. From start position, flexed legs are drawn up until the pelvis can be supported with the hands. The arms are flexed 90 degrees at the elbows, the upper arms resting on the floor. From this stable position, the knees are slowly extended overhead. Gradual stretching of hamstring muscles is achieved with the lumbar spine in the safe flexed position and protected from torsional force. (C) Knee-Flexion Sit-Up. Sit-up is performed with knees flexed, no fixation of the feet, and no lunging with upper body or arms.

lengthy discussion of degenerative disc disease, his most probable diagnosis, and its future consequences. Such educational approaches, which are vital in the treatment of chronic or recurrent low back pain, are usually deferred until the patient has had several attacks and has begun to recognize the long term nature and serious implications of the condition.

Chronic Low Back Pain

Whereas acute low back pain is commonly treated mainly or exclusively by occupational physicians and nurses, chronic low back troubles usually come under the care of outside physicians or other treatment facilities. There are, however, a number of vital functions in the treatment of chronic low back pain which can often best be fulfilled by the occupational physician or nurse.

If the symptoms are job-related in any way, the first contact with the patient may be made in the plant medical department and the initial evaluation performed there. After completion of the first examination, time should be set aside to discuss the findings thoroughly with the patient and begin the lengthy but rewarding process of patient education. This can best be done, in unhurried fashion, by the original examiner. If the probable diagnosis is degenerative disc disease in one of its several phases, the pathomechanics and natural life history of the condition should be explained, using diagrams similar to those in figure 45 and the patient's own x-rays as illustrative material. Such explanations, being simple and mechanically-derived, are usually well understood and accepted. Offering rational explanation for disturbing and frightening symptoms, they are occasionally the only treatment which is necessary. In the patient who will require outside specialist care, valuable ground-work is laid for what may lie ahead. In either case, an important one-on-one relationship has been established between the patient and a medical person closely connected with the workplace. This relationship is of inestimable value and may be the single most important factor in determining the outcome of treatment and management.

In the modern medical world of specialism, highly technical diagnostic procedures and group care, there is often no one to talk to the patient. The average low back patient, suffering a condition which is painful, alarming and inherently evocative of powerful psychological reaction, stands in desperate need of an omsbudsperson to provide support, explain diagnostic findings, discuss proposed treatment and correlate rehabilitative efforts. The occupational physician or nurse may be ideally cast in this supportive and interpretative role, operating with one foot in the medical world, the other in the workplace, and out of a close and caring relationship with the patient.

Close liason between the occupational physician or nurse and outside diagnostic and treatment facilities must be maintained if the patient is to make an optimal recovery. The outside physician usually knows little of the work situation, apart from the often inaccurate information imparted by the patient, and the opportunity for an early return to modified work may be missed simply by lack of communication.

It is important that regular contact be maintained with the patient by the supervisor and other appropriate company representatives simply as a demonstration of concern. The feeling on the part of patients that the employer does not care is a common element in disability determination.

MANAGEMENT

If the proposition is accepted that most backache in industry is episodic, recurrent, unrelated to injury as ordinarily defined, and largely unpreventable; and, if it is recognized that most common types of backache are not amenable to specific treatment which will effect cure, then the prime objective of management is to control disability. Low back disability in industry is a social as well as a medical problem, its degree and duration often determined as much by socio-economic factors as by the severity of the disease.

Effective control of low back disability in industry requires the dedication and cooperation of the entire industrial establishment from top management on down, and cannot be accomplished by the medical department alone. Prerequisite to the committment of the organization is knowledge, both of the epidemiological scope of the problem, and of the typical clinical manifestations. Few problems of this magnitude are so cluttered with misinformation. Medical people in industry must spearhead a broad-based educational effort which is the foundation of effective control of disability, both in the working population as a whole and at the individual patient level.

Even such seemingly important information as the total annual dollar cost of low back disability is not fully known in most industries. Costs for Workers' Compensation cases are well documented, but are often assumed to represent the total pay-out. Some states, however, mandate the payment of disability benefits for non work-related illnesses and injury and the cost of low back disability, which ranks consistently among the top conditions in this category, is generally much less well known. Many companies have plans for the indemnification of long term disability, extending the state-mandated period for non work-related conditions and supplementing payments made under Workers' Compensation schedules. Because most patients with low back disability become eligible for Long Term Disability plans at a relatively early age with a condition which seldom threatens longevity, the roles of such indemnity plans carry an ever increasing number of low back patients. The direct cost of low back disability to industry is the sum of the amounts expended under each of the three plans. The indirect costs are probably incalculable. They would include such items as disrupted production schedules, the training of replacement workers, creation of make-work situations and the dollars and man hours expended in attempts to prevent low back pain at work. Once all the figures are collected and estimated, low back trouble is likely to emerge as Industry's most expensive medical problem.

In addition to cost analysis, it is important that all persons in the workplace who may interface with the patient in any capacity have a working knowledge of the true causes and typical clinical manifestations of backache. This, to prevent the man-made barriers to recovery which arise from longheld biases and anecdotal misinformation concerning the nature of backache at work and the attitudinal postures which result from them.

Since it has been demonstrated that long term disability back cases account for the major share of the high costs, it becomes axiomatic that the potential high cost cases be identified early and that effective means of prompt intervention be instituted if control is to be effected.

Identification

Early identification of the potential long term disability back patient requires, in addition to the best obtainable knowledge of the low back condition, a perceptive assessment of the whole patient, physically and psychologicaly, and familiarity with both the work and the home environments. Disability is usually determined by a complex mosaic of factors, many of which have little to do with the condition in the low back. Table 5 lists some of the more common risk factors which may serve as warning signals of potential long term disability problems.

RISK FACTORS FOR PROLONGED LOW BACK DISABILITY

A. The Patient
1. Limited vocational assets (age, physical condition, education)
2. Poor work record. Job dissatisfaction
3. Frequent visits to medical department for minor complaints
4. Frequent absences from work for minor conditions
5. Language barrier

B. The History of Injury
1. Exaggerated severity of injury incident. Blames others.
2. Anger toward Company or its representatives
3. Dramatic description of symptoms
4. Inappropriate symptoms
5. Past history of disabling low back pain, myelogram, surgery

C. The Physical Examination
1. Over-reaction to examination maneuvers
2. Inappropriate and inconsistent areas of tenderness
3. Differences in findings when distracted or believed unobserved
4. Complaint of severe aggravation of symptoms by the examination

D. The Worksite
1. Heavy work. Limited opportunity for modified job, transfer
2. Inflexible, demanding supervision. Bias concerning backache
3. Patient not popular with supervisors or co-workers
4. Inappropriate benefit structure

E. The Home
1. Over-protective spouse
2. Back disability useful in coping with marital problems
3. Back disability useful in coping with parenting problems

F. The Course of Treatment
1. Frequent changes of primary therapist
2. Care in charge of inappropriate therapists
3. Multiple consultations by physicians in same specialty
4. Disparagement of therapists
5. Visits to hospital emergency department with low back symptoms
6. More than two surgeries

Table 5. Risk Factors for Prolonged Low Back Disability

Intervention

The fact that about 85 percent of all low back incidents either cause no lost time from work or result in short term disabilities of three weeks or less implies that the intervention process need not be universally employed. It suggests, however, that active intervention should be triggered by any absence with low back pain exceeding four to six weeks in cases where no definite date for return to work has been established.

Effective steps in intervention are derived for each individual case from careful appraisal of the risk factors at play. Most potential long term disability patients will have several risk factors, some of which may be partly or wholly remediable, some of which may not. The aim in the intervention process is to so reduce the total load of risk factors as to allow the earliest possible return to productive activity. The rapidly diminishing return rate with the passage of each month of disability stresses the need for moving decisively, once the intervention process has been initiated.

The details of implementation of the process will vary from company to company in accordance with the numbers and types of medical and paramedical personnel available. Where commercial Workers' Compensation Insurance carriers are involved, intervention is often carried out mainly by their personnel. In general, the process is most successful when it is organized and administered by one individual, ideally the physician or nurse from the Company who knows the patient best. Additional information and advice in the various segments of the complex pattern may have to be sought from others. Details concerning the home environment, for instance, can often be furnished by the visiting nurse, if there is one, or by a supervisor or group leader who calls upon the patient at home. Normally, worksite information is obtained from the supervisor, but there may be instances in which this information must be obtained from others. Liason with outside treatment facilities is usually best established by the area physician or the medical director, but the occupational nurse may be just as effective in certain circumstances. In general, the salient facts and opinions are collected from an informal team, which may be different for each patient, and the practical steps in intervention are agreed upon. Patient contact is handled by one individual, judged by the members of the team to be most effective.

Implementation obviously requires cooperation throughout the organization, and this implies both dedication of top management and a sizeable cadre of individuals in many areas of the company who are knowledgeable about low back problems.

General Measures

In addition to the efforts directed toward the individual low back patient who has been identified as being at high risk for long term disability, certain measures of a more general nature, instituted plant wide, are effective in minimizing low back disability. Much remains to be accomplished in the field of job and workplace design to make it possible for more workers to perfom more jobs, more days, with mild to moderate impairments. Such steps will probably have little effect upon the incidence of low back pain, but they are important in controlling low back disability.

There is great need for company sponsorship and supervision of a rehabilitative exercise program for patients with low back pain who have been off the job for periods of three weeks or more, especially if they are returning to physically demanding work. Weakness and atrophy of the supportive muscles of the trunk occurs very rapidly during the period of enforced rest imposed by back pain and, unless these people are physically reconditioned, they are very likely to have recurrent problems shortly after returning to work.

Some companies have had success with general physical fitness programs. While it is often true that those most likely to benefit from exercise programs are least likely to participate, any approach which will raise general levels of fitness is likely to minimize disability from low back pain. This was born out in a 20 year study of low back disability among 1500 working men. Those who carried out a regular exercise program and returned to normal levels of physical activity experienced as many attacks of low back pain as the more sedentary, but handled each attack better and lost significantly less time from work.

Low back schools are currently popular. For patients who have had low back trouble, they seem to play a valuable role in disability control so long as they do not replace the continuing one-on-one relationship between the patient and the primary therapist. The worker who has had little or no problem with the back is unlikely to be much interested in back schools and their role in preventing backache is doubtful.

It may be appropriate for companies to review their disability benefit plans. Inappropriate benefit packages occasionally result in the patient having a larger after-tax income while disabled then would be earned by working. Figuring in this determination, in addition to company benefits, are such items as Social Security disability payments, foregiveness of mortgage and installment debt payment during disability and the income from privately held disability insurance policies. It may be reasonable to evaluate the total disability income from all sources for each patient and tailor the company program accordingly. Rehabilitation attempts are likely to be fruitless in most cases if it costs the patient money to return to work.

Summary

The high costs of low back trouble can be reduced significantly and workers better served by directing the efforts of the organization toward minimizing disability rather than concentrating on the prevention of low back injury, which has been the theme of the past fifty fruitless years. Low back injury, at least in the sense in which injury is generally understood, accounts for less than five percent of chronic low back problems likely to have long term disability. Nearly 70 percent of problem cases have a degenerative condition which, at the present time, is neither preventable nor curable. Degenerative disc disease, while it may account for a working lifetime of episodic and recurrent backache, is not inherently nor even very frequently disabling. When prolonged disability does occur, the low back condition may be only the socially acceptable label for a complex pattern of intertwined difficulties which really determine disability. Understanding the true situation and remedying those problems which are solvable will result not only in the saving of dollars, but, very often, in the salvation of a human being.

INDEX

A
Abdominal muscle exercises, 151, 152, Fig. 47, Fig. 48
Achilles tendon rupture, 115, 116
Acromio-clavicular joint injuries, 69-71
Acute low back pain
    clinical picture, 146, 147
    diagnosis, 147-149
    examination, 163
    exercise, 151, 152, Fig. 47
    pain-spasm reflex, 150, 151
    physiotherapy, 151
    traction, 152, Fig. 47
    treatment, 150-154
    x-ray, 147
Aggravation, pre-existing condition, 6, 149
Anatomy
    see Contents; Structure and Function for specific area
Ankle
    anatomy, 85-87, Fig. 30, Fig. 31
    contusions, 95
    fractures
        eversion-external rotation, 91-95, Fig. 35
        inversion-internal rotation, 91, Fig. 34
    sprains
        mild, 87, 88
        severe, 88-90, Fig. 32, Fig. 33
Anterior compartment syndrome, 116, 117
Arches of foot, 73,
Avascular necrosis
    carpal navicular, 46, 47
    femoral neck, 120
Avulsion fractures, general, 15
    base of fith metatarsal, 77, Fig. 24

N

S